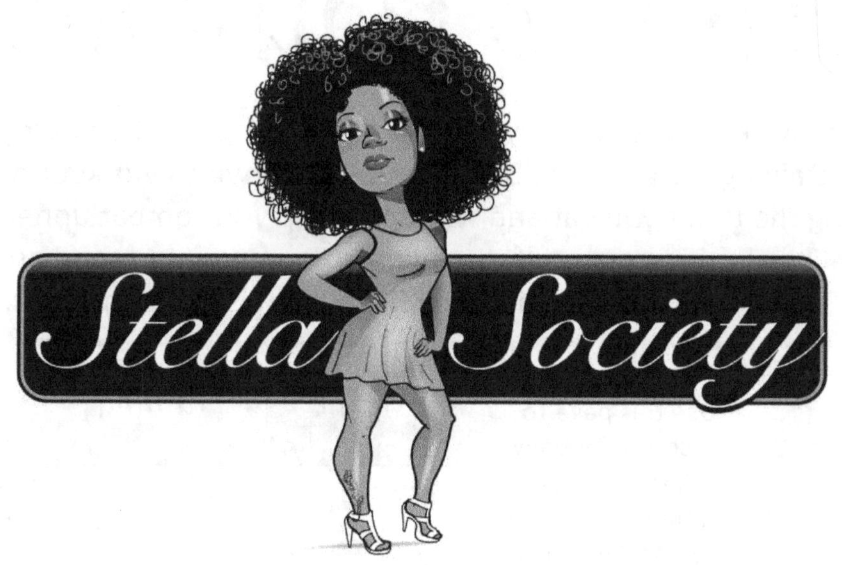

Thank you for participating in the Stella Project 2.0, a 40 day fitness confidence and nutrition challenge.
If you purchased this journal and you are not a member of the Stella Project, no worries. You can find us at stellasocietyacademy dot com, or just use it on your own 40 day fitness journey.

Always consult a physician before beginning an exercise program.

How to use your journal

Journaling has many benefits especially when tracking progress. Recording your thoughts before training can help you better understand why a workout did or didn't go too well. Recalling the times you eat and what can help you combat unnecessary cravings. Journaling also increases self-discipline, improves your mood and boost comprehension. Please use this journal to aid in your goals through your 40 days.

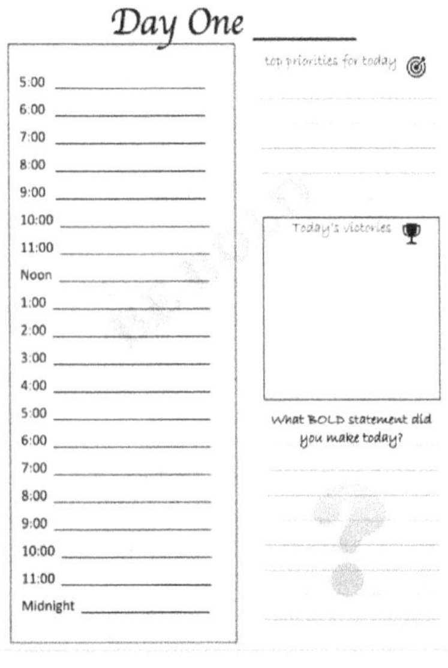

Use this page to record your daily schedule, meals, training, meetings, etc. Make sure you put the date. List your top priorities hat must be completed that day. Record your victories, like drinking all your water and reflect on the daily bestellatude

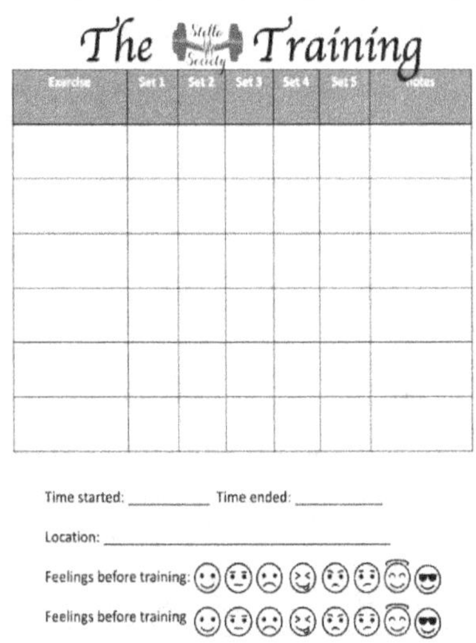

Use this page to record your training sessions. Write them down ahead of time and watch the video in case you have questions. Put the time your started and completed the training as well as how you felt before and after. Leave a note as to why you felt a certain before the training. This could effect how it went.

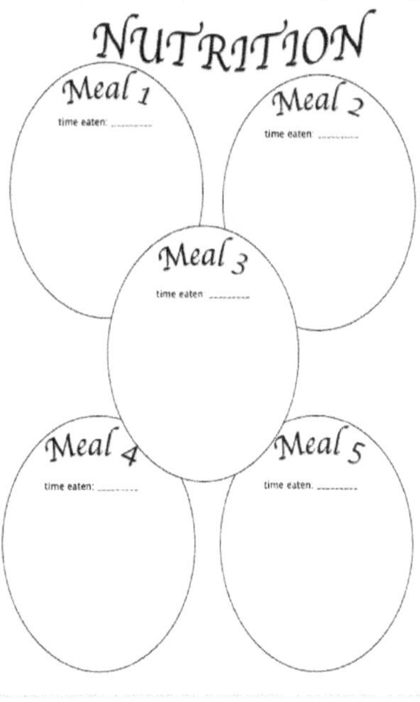

Use this page to record your meals and the time you ate them. This is important especially when tracking your progress. Try to eat your meals at the same time each day. Get your machine on a schedule so it knows how to operate its fuel.

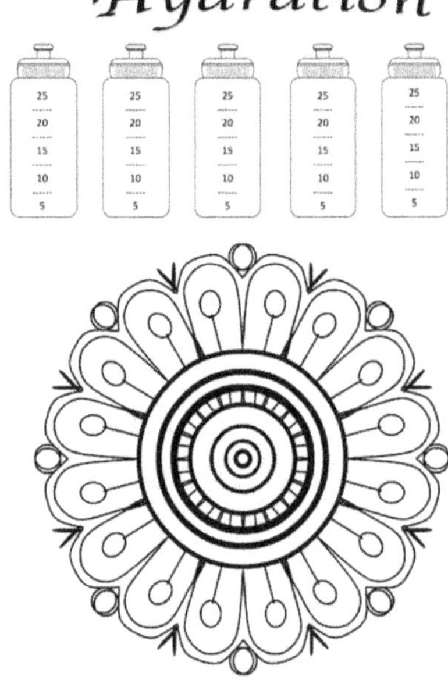

Use this page to record your water intake. Color the bottles as you complete each one. Also each hydration page has a mandala graphic to color. Coloring is a form of meditation. Choose to color this instead of reaching for something to snack on that's not you're your meal plan.

R.O.S.E.S GOAL

Rationale – why are you participating in this 40 day challenge?

____

____

Objective – what do you look to accomplish during the 40 days? What is the end game, goal?

____

____

Strategy – how will you go about completing your objective? What actions will you take.

____

____

Evaluation – how and when will you evaluate you progress? Will you use inches, weight, look, or clothes?

____

____

Schedule – create a schedule for the next 40 days. Include anything that will get in the way of your goal and find a work around.

____

____

Measurements

DATE: ___________

Weight: _______

Neck _______

Shoulders _______

Chest _______

Bicep / upper arm left _______ right _______

Forearm left _______ right _______

Waist _______

Hips _______

Thighs left _______ right _______

Calf left _______ right _______

Only I Can Change My Life, No One Can Do It For Me

Day One _______

<table>
<tr><td>

5:00 _______________________

6:00 _______________________

7:00 _______________________

8:00 _______________________

9:00 _______________________

10:00 ______________________

11:00 ______________________

Noon ______________________

1:00 _______________________

2:00 _______________________

3:00 _______________________

4:00 _______________________

5:00 _______________________

6:00 _______________________

7:00 _______________________

8:00 _______________________

9:00 _______________________

10:00 ______________________

11:00 ______________________

Midnight _________________

</td><td>

top priorities for today 🎯

____

____

____

____

Today's victories 🏆

What BOLD statement did you make today?

____

____

____

____

____

____

</td></tr>
</table>

The Training

Exercise	Set 1	Set 2	Set 3	Set 4	Set 5	notes

Time started: ________________ Time ended: ________________

Location: ____

Feelings before training: 😊 😐 ☹️ 😜 😠 😟 😊 😎

Feelings after training 😊 😐 ☹️ 😜 😠 😟 😊 😎

NUTRITION

Meal 1
time eaten: _________

Meal 2
time eaten: _________

Meal 3
time eaten: _________

Meal 4
time eaten: _________

Meal 5
time eaten: _________

Hydration

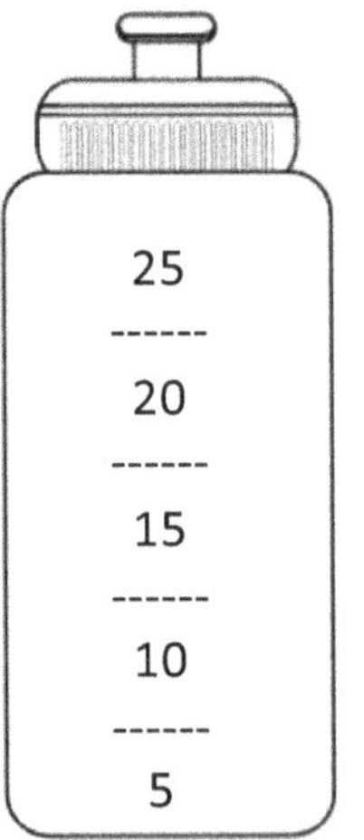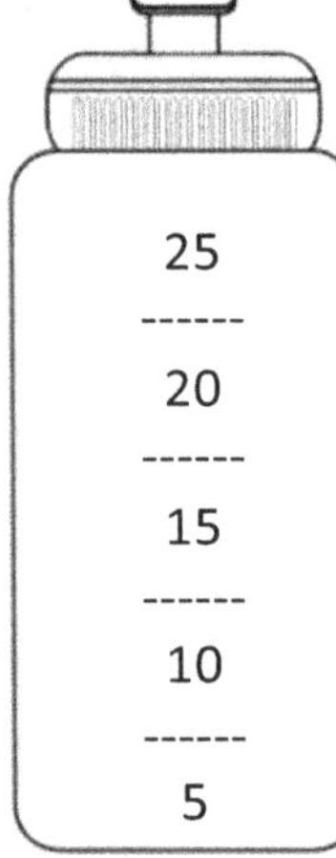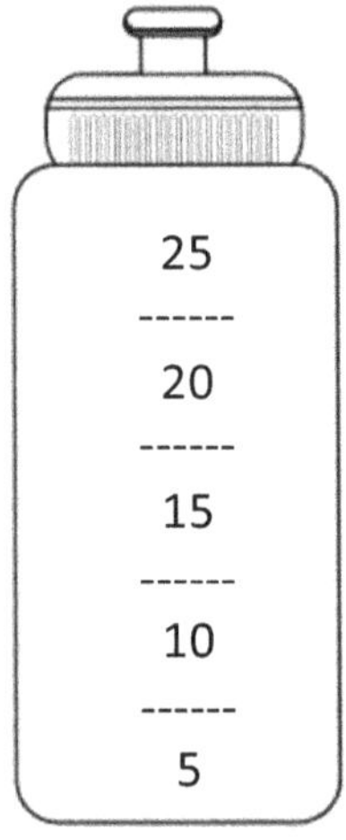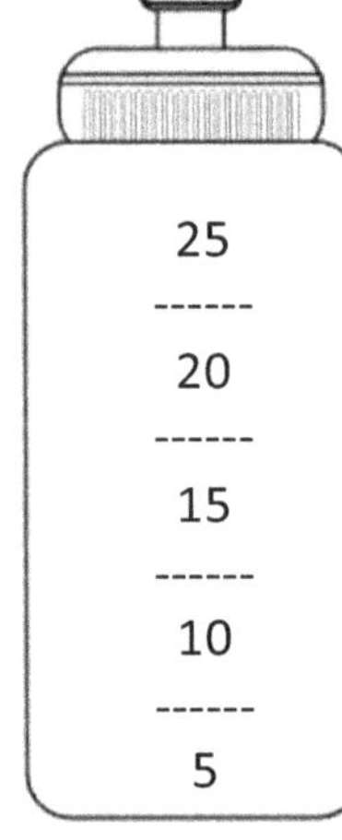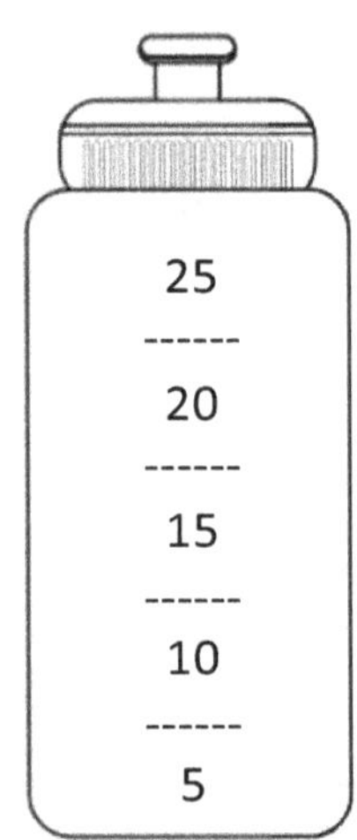

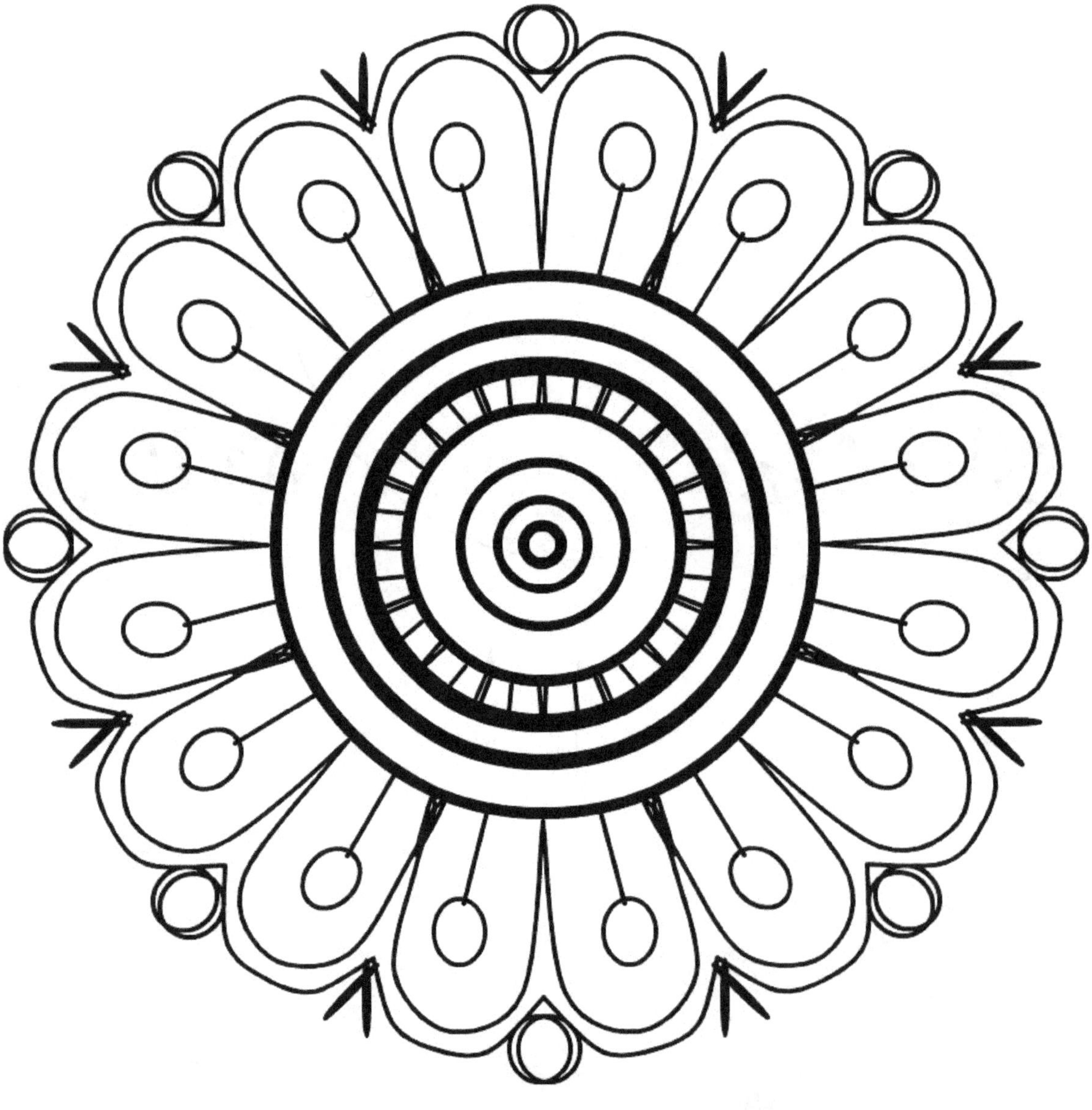

Day Two _______

Time	
5:00	____________________
6:00	____________________
7:00	____________________
8:00	____________________
9:00	____________________
10:00	____________________
11:00	____________________
Noon	____________________
1:00	____________________
2:00	____________________
3:00	____________________
4:00	____________________
5:00	____________________
6:00	____________________
7:00	____________________
8:00	____________________
9:00	____________________
10:00	____________________
11:00	____________________
Midnight	____________________

top priorities for today

____
____
____
____

Today's victories

What is one thing that makes you unique??

____
____
____
____
____
____
____

The Training

Exercise	Set 1	Set 2	Set 3	Set 4	Set 5	notes

Time started: _____________ Time ended: _____________

Location: ____

Feelings before training:

Feelings after training

NUTRITION

Meal 1

time eaten: _________

Meal 2

time eaten: _________

Meal 3

time eaten: _________

Meal 4

time eaten: _________

Meal 5

time eaten: _________

Hydration

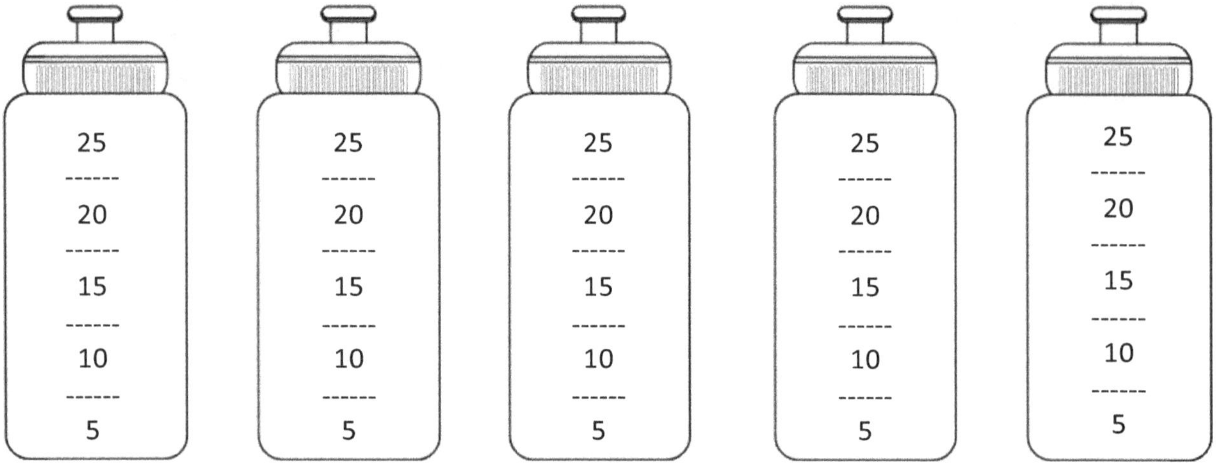

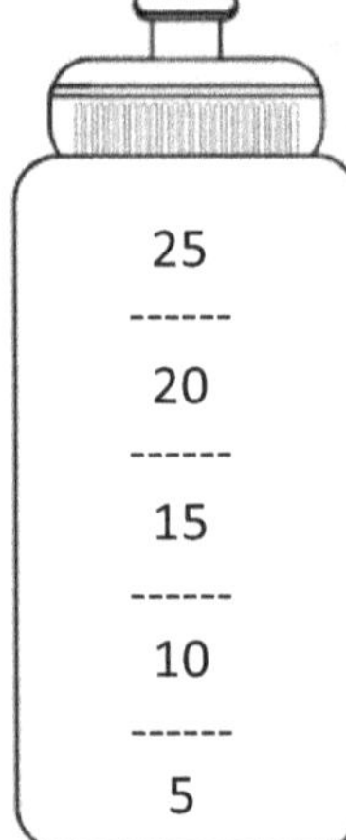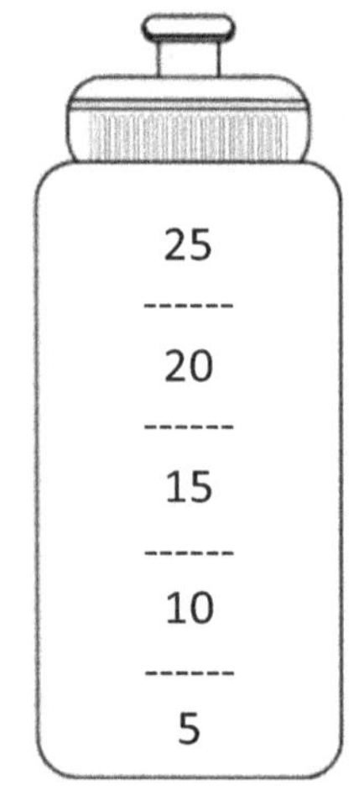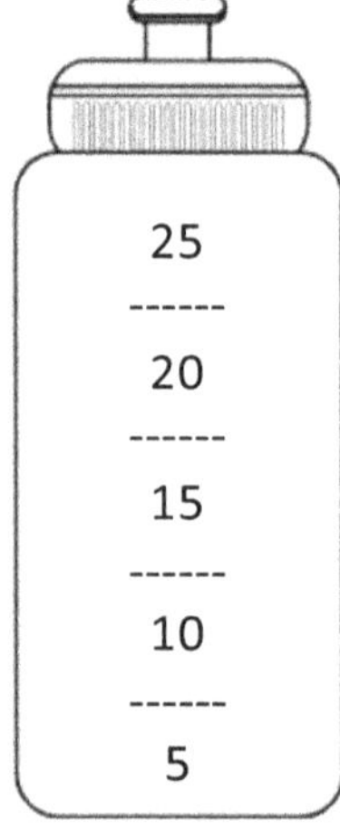

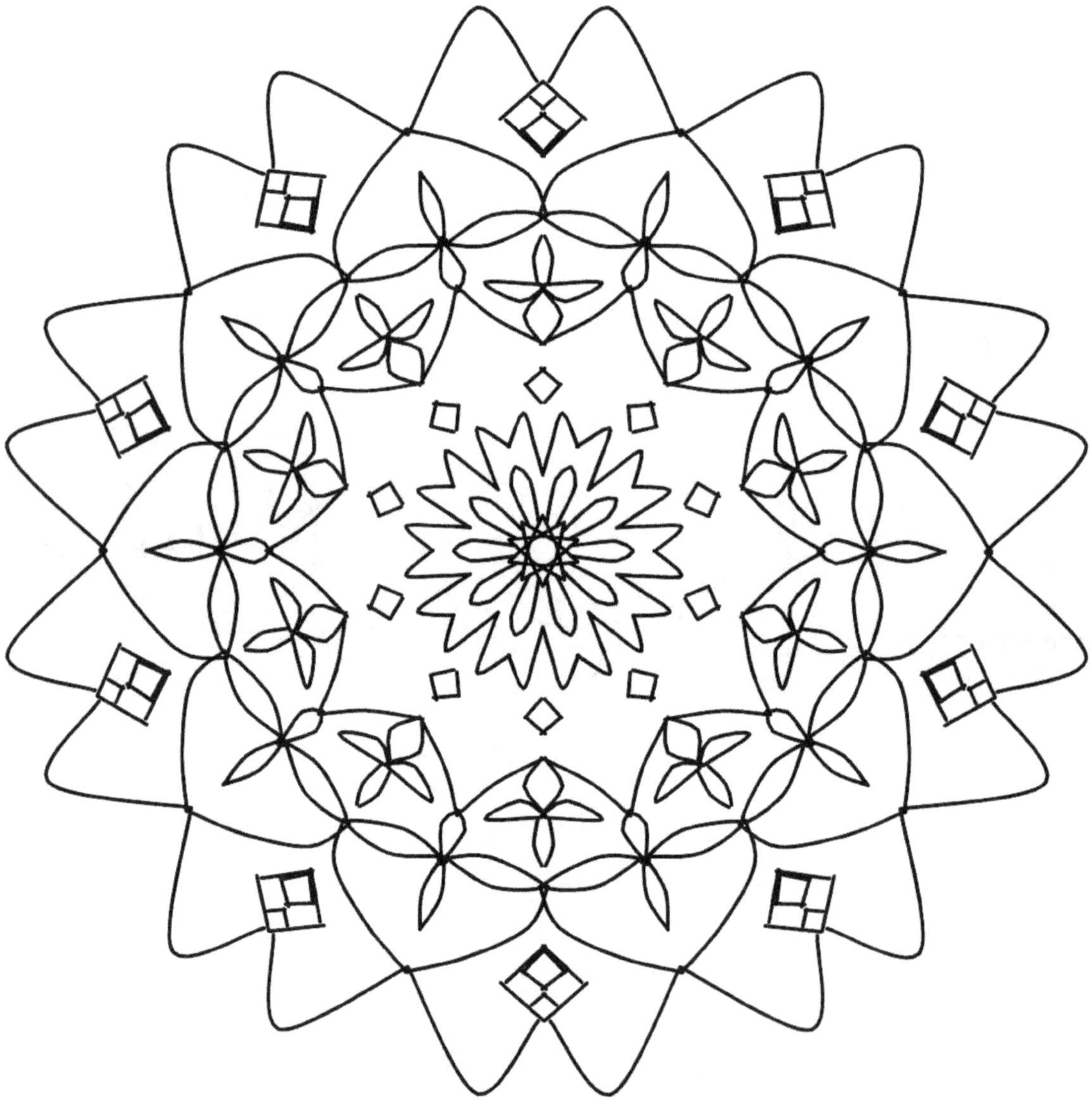

Day Three ______

5:00 ____________________	

5:00 ____________________

6:00 ____________________

7:00 ____________________

8:00 ____________________

9:00 ____________________

10:00 ____________________

11:00 ____________________

Noon ____________________

1:00 ____________________

2:00 ____________________

3:00 ____________________

4:00 ____________________

5:00 ____________________

6:00 ____________________

7:00 ____________________

8:00 ____________________

9:00 ____________________

10:00 ____________________

11:00 ____________________

Midnight ____________________

top priorities for today

Today's victories

What makes you brave?

The Stella Society Training

Exercise	Set 1	Set 2	Set 3	Set 4	Set 5	notes

Time started: _____________ Time ended: _______________

Location: ____

Feelings before training: 🙂 😐 ☹️ 😜 😠 😕 😊 😎

Feelings after training 🙂 😐 ☹️ 😜 😠 😕 😊 😎

NUTRITION

Meal 1

time eaten: _________

Meal 2

time eaten: _________

Meal 3

time eaten: _________

Meal 4

time eaten: _________

Meal 5

time eaten: _________

Hydration

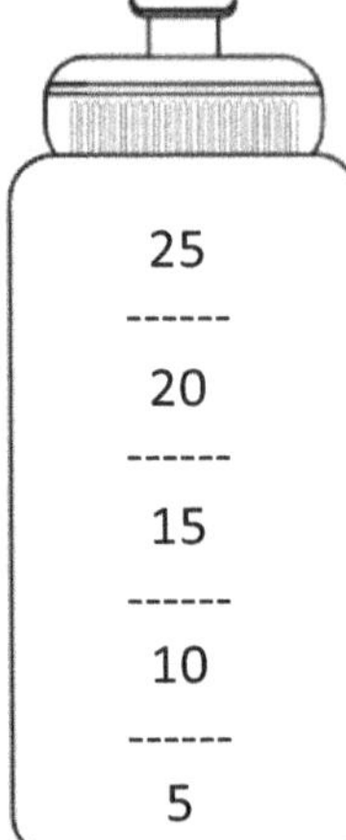

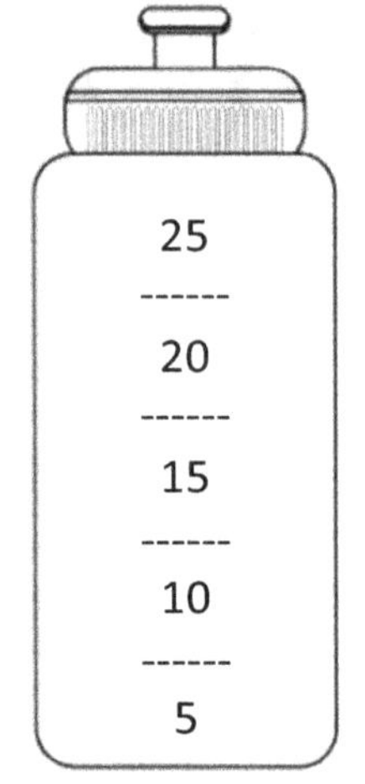

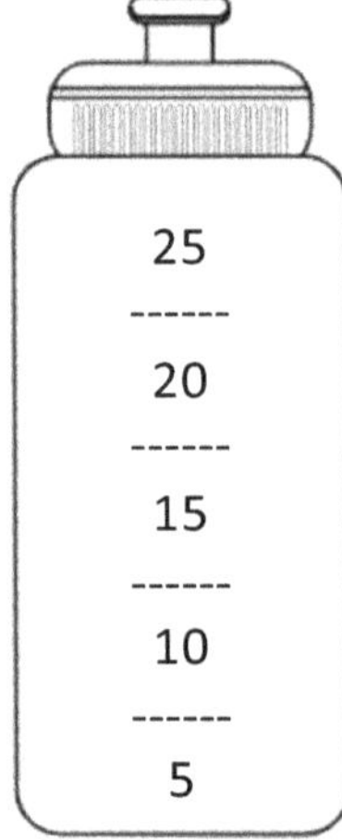

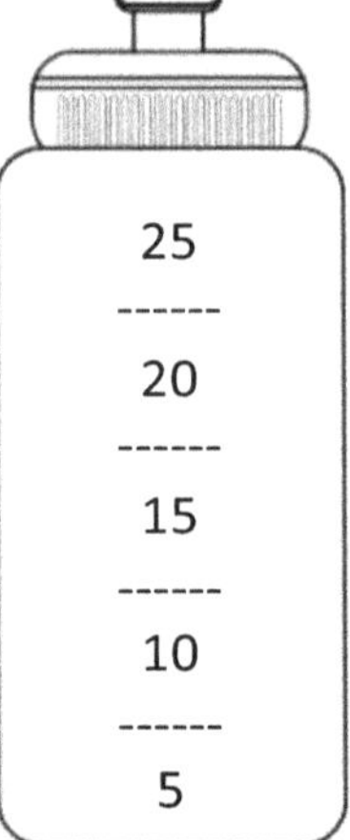

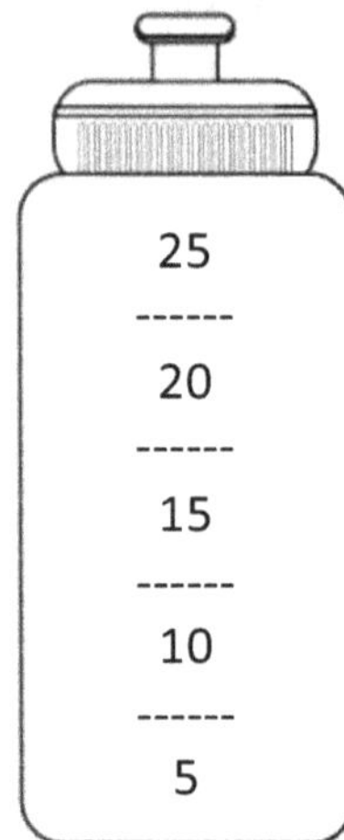

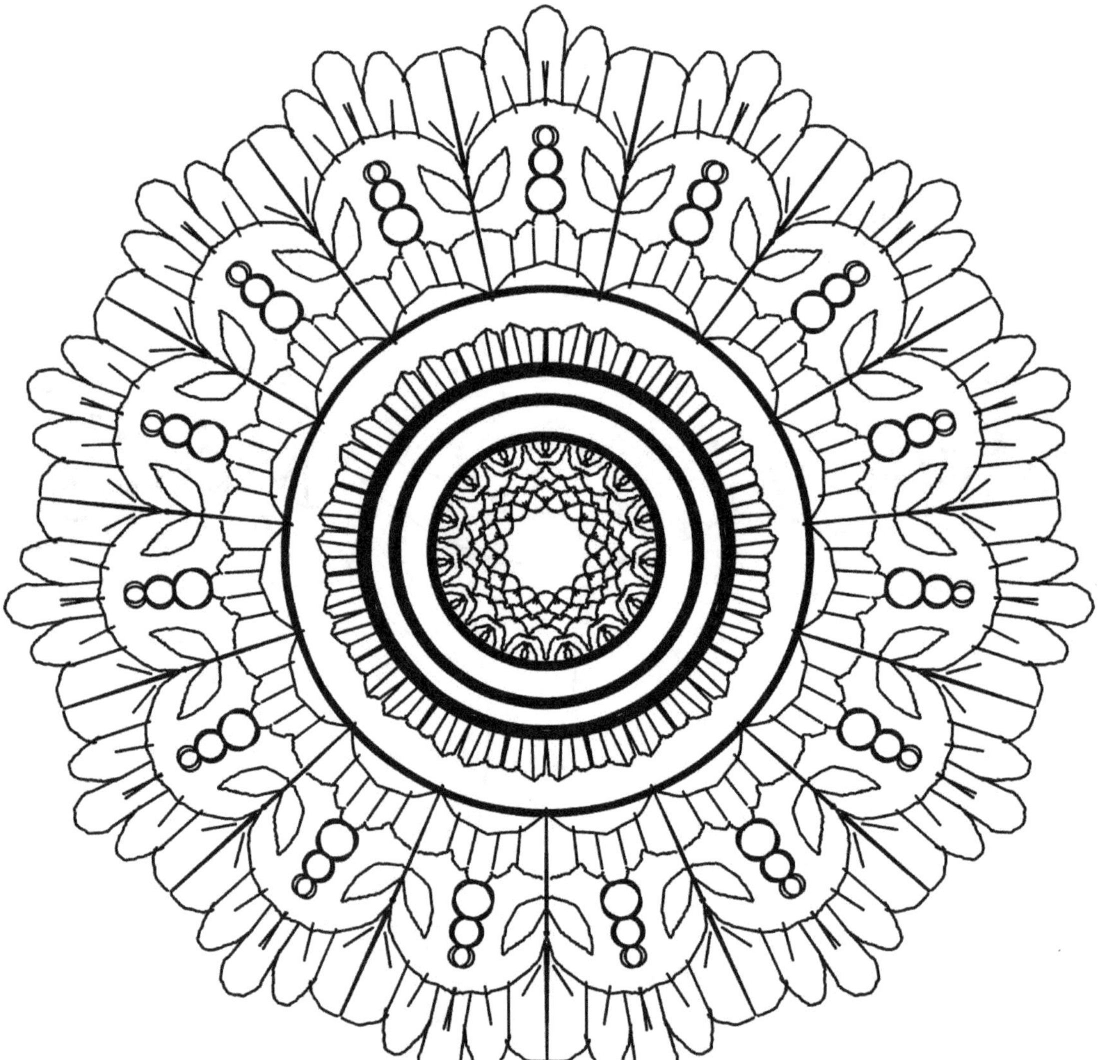

Day Four _______

5:00 _______________	top priorities for today 🎯

5:00 ______________________

6:00 ______________________

7:00 ______________________

8:00 ______________________

9:00 ______________________

10:00 ____________________

11:00 ____________________

Noon _____________________

1:00 ______________________

2:00 ______________________

3:00 ______________________

4:00 ______________________

5:00 ______________________

6:00 ______________________

7:00 ______________________

8:00 ______________________

9:00 ______________________

10:00 ____________________

11:00 ____________________

Midnight _________________

top priorities for today 🎯

Today's victories 🏆

What did you commit to today that will make for a better tomorrow?

The Training

Exercise	Set 1	Set 2	Set 3	Set 4	Set 5	notes

Time started: _____________ Time ended: _______________

Location: ____

Feelings before training:

Feelings aftertraining

NUTRITION

Meal 1
time eaten: _________

Meal 2
time eaten: _________

Meal 3
time eaten: _________

Meal 4
time eaten: _________

Meal 5
time eaten: _________

Hydration

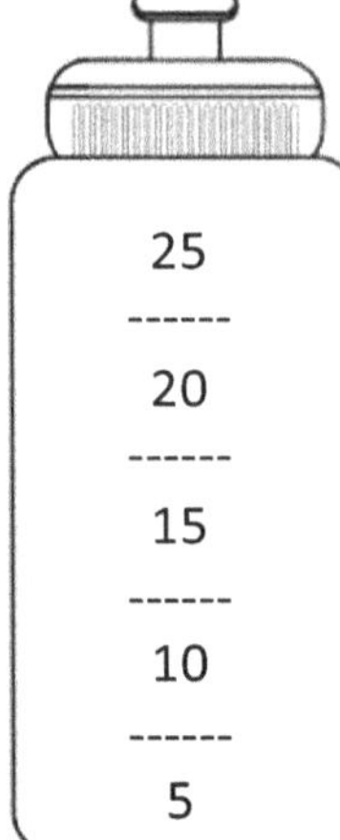

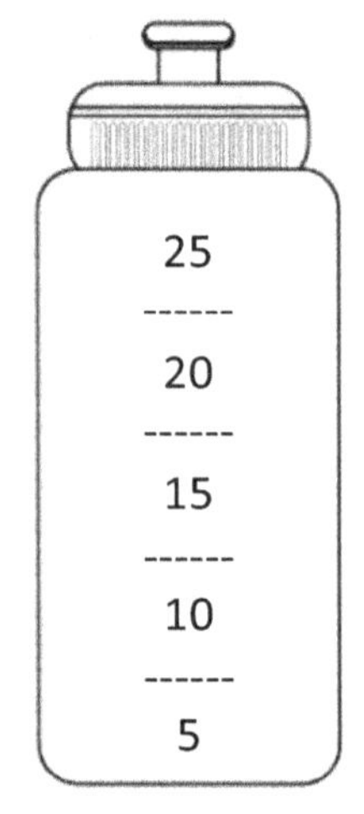

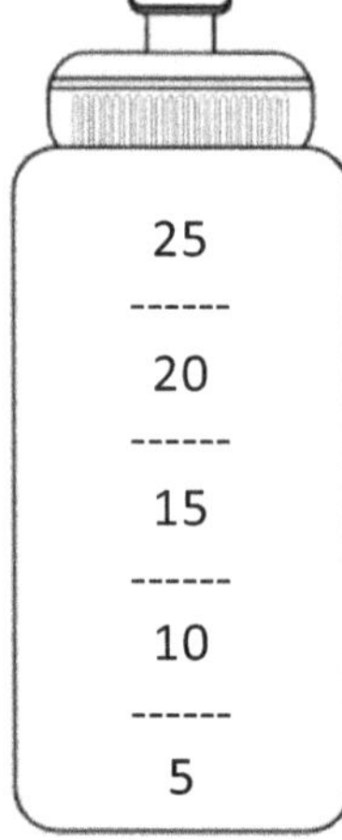

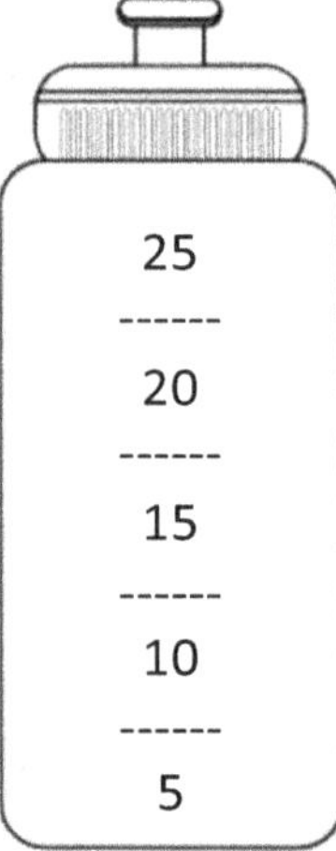

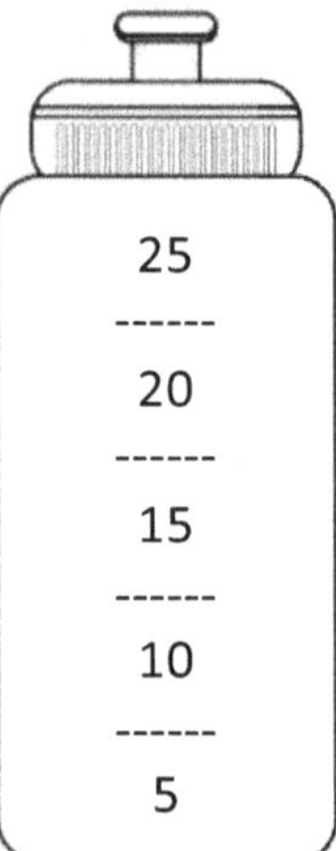

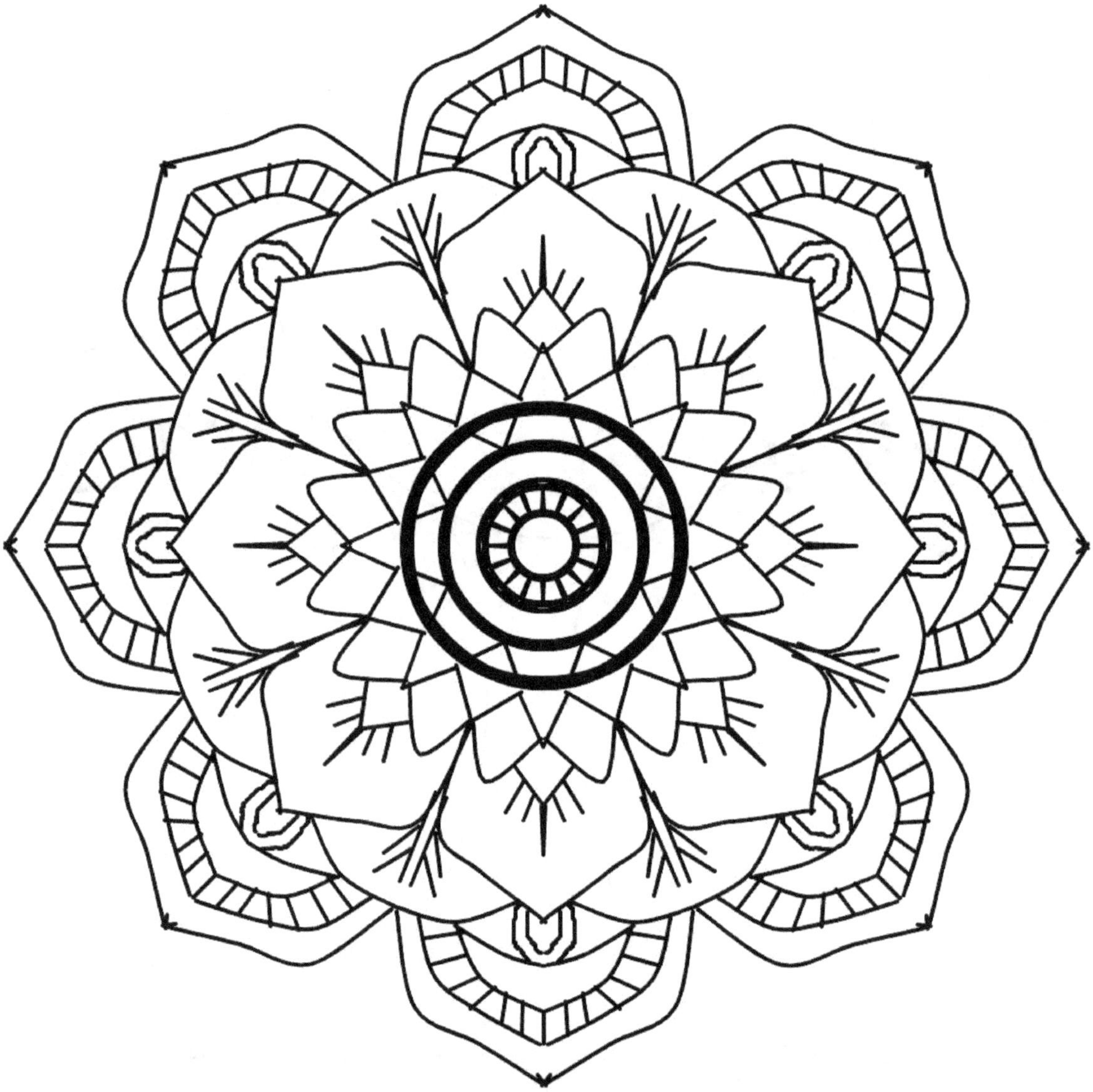

Day Five _______

5:00	_____________________
6:00	_____________________
7:00	_____________________
8:00	_____________________
9:00	_____________________
10:00	_____________________
11:00	_____________________
Noon	_____________________
1:00	_____________________
2:00	_____________________
3:00	_____________________
4:00	_____________________
5:00	_____________________
6:00	_____________________
7:00	_____________________
8:00	_____________________
9:00	_____________________
10:00	_____________________
11:00	_____________________
Midnight	_____________________

top priorities for today 

____
____
____
____
____

Today's victories

Who is the wisest person you know?
Talk to them today.

____
____
____
____
____
____

The Training

Exercise	Set 1	Set 2	Set 3	Set 4	Set 5	notes

Time started: _____________   Time ended: _______________

Location: ____

Feelings before training:

Feelings after training

NUTRITION

Meal 1
time eaten: _________

Meal 2
time eaten: _________

Meal 3
time eaten: _________

Meal 4
time eaten: _________

Meal 5
time eaten: _________

Hydration

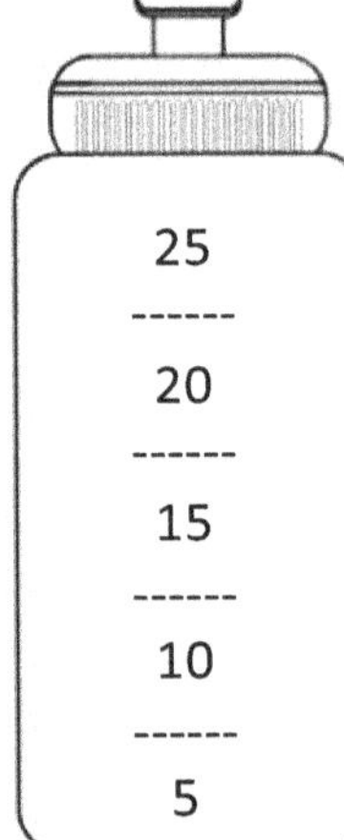

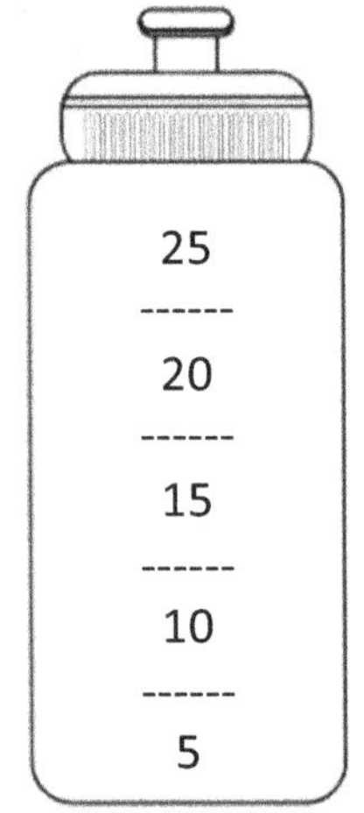

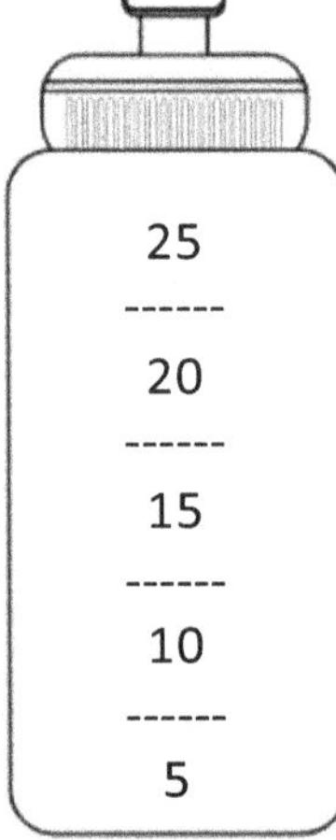

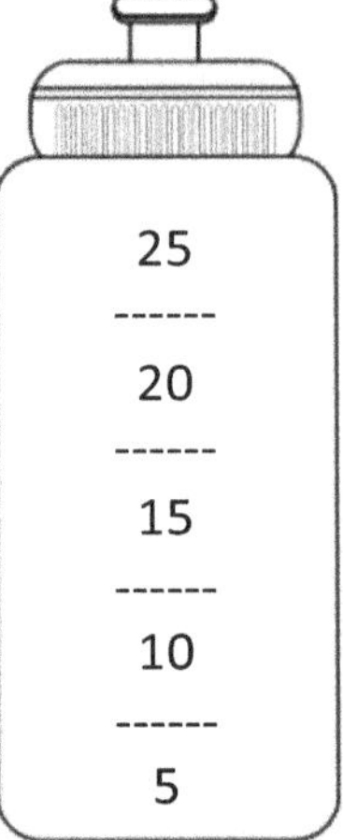

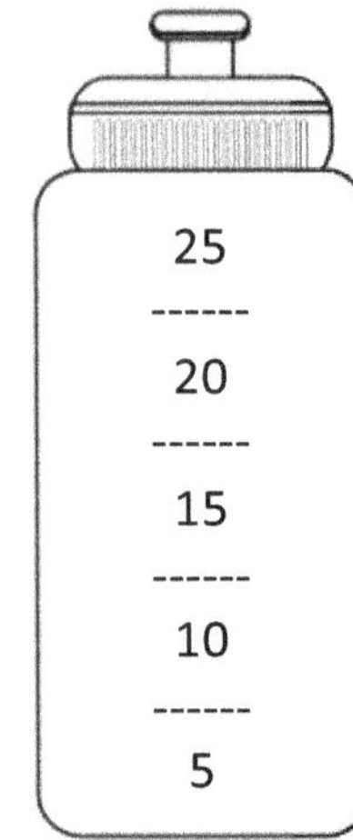

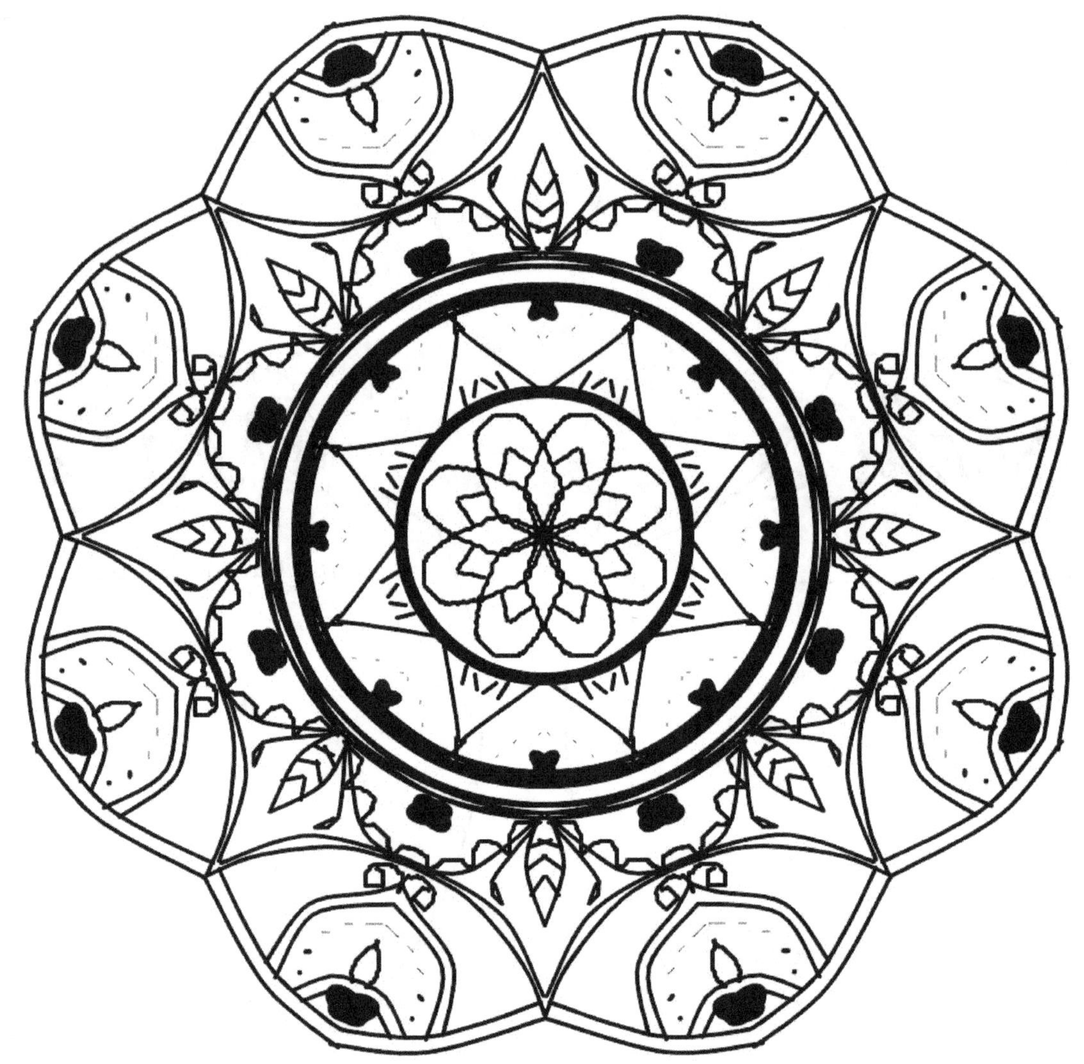

Day Six _______

<table>
<tr><td>

5:00 ____________________

6:00 ____________________

7:00 ____________________

8:00 ____________________

9:00 ____________________

10:00 ___________________

11:00 ___________________

Noon ____________________

1:00 ____________________

2:00 ____________________

3:00 ____________________

4:00 ____________________

5:00 ____________________

6:00 ____________________

7:00 ____________________

8:00 ____________________

9:00 ____________________

10:00 ___________________

11:00 ___________________

Midnight _________________

</td><td>

top priorities for today 

____

____

____

____

____

Today's victories 🏆

What is your biggest fear and how do you get over it?

____

____

____

____

____

____

</td></tr>
</table>

The *Stella Society* Training

Exercise	Set 1	Set 2	Set 3	Set 4	Set 5	notes

Time started: _______________   Time ended: _______________

Location: ____

Feelings before training:

Feelings after training

NUTRITION

Meal 1
time eaten: _________

Meal 2
time eaten: _________

Meal 3
time eaten: _________

Meal 4
time eaten: _________

Meal 5
time eaten: _________

Hydration

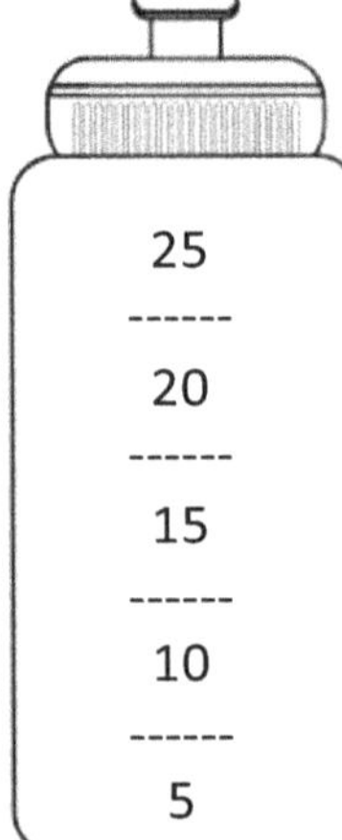

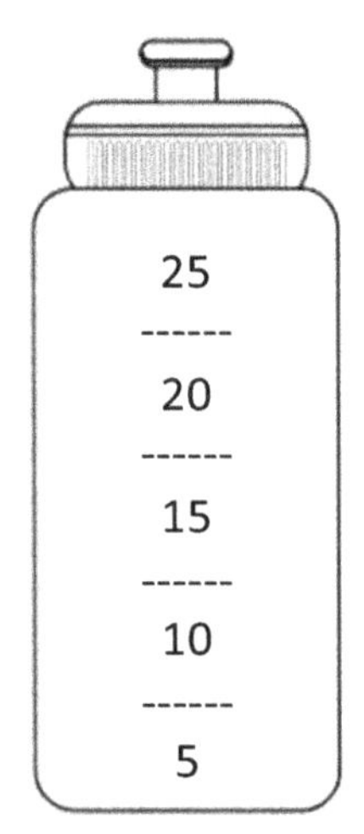

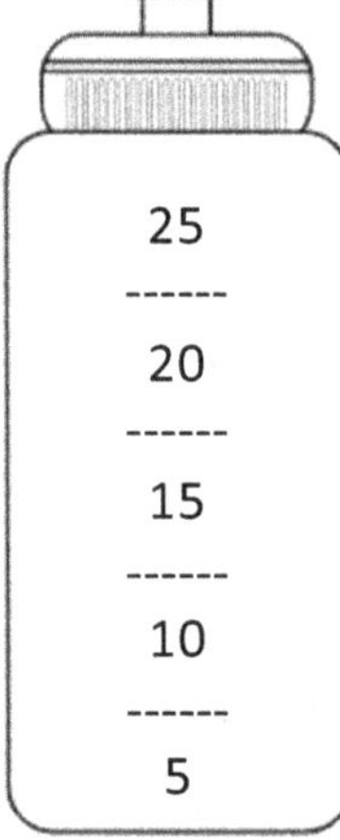

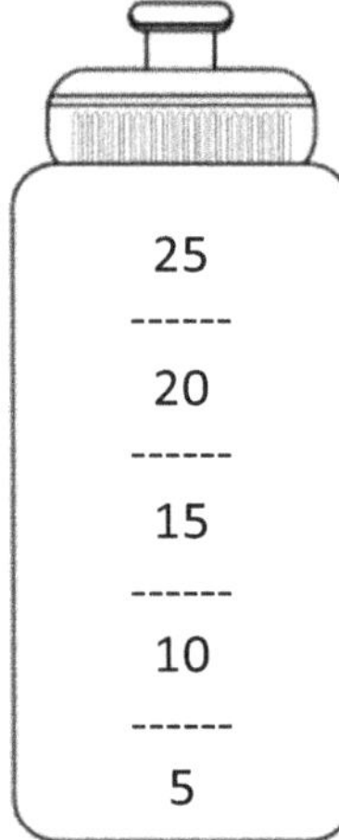

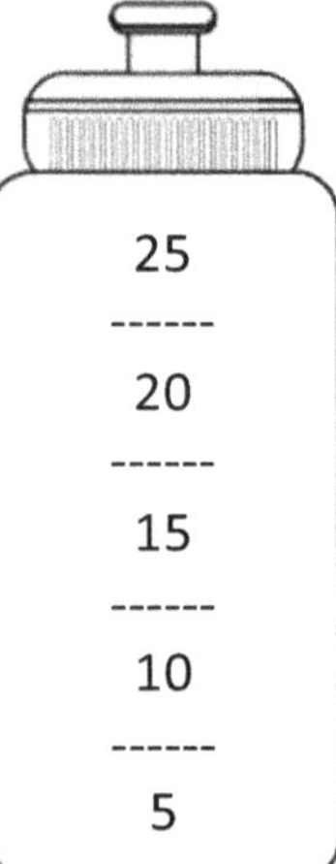

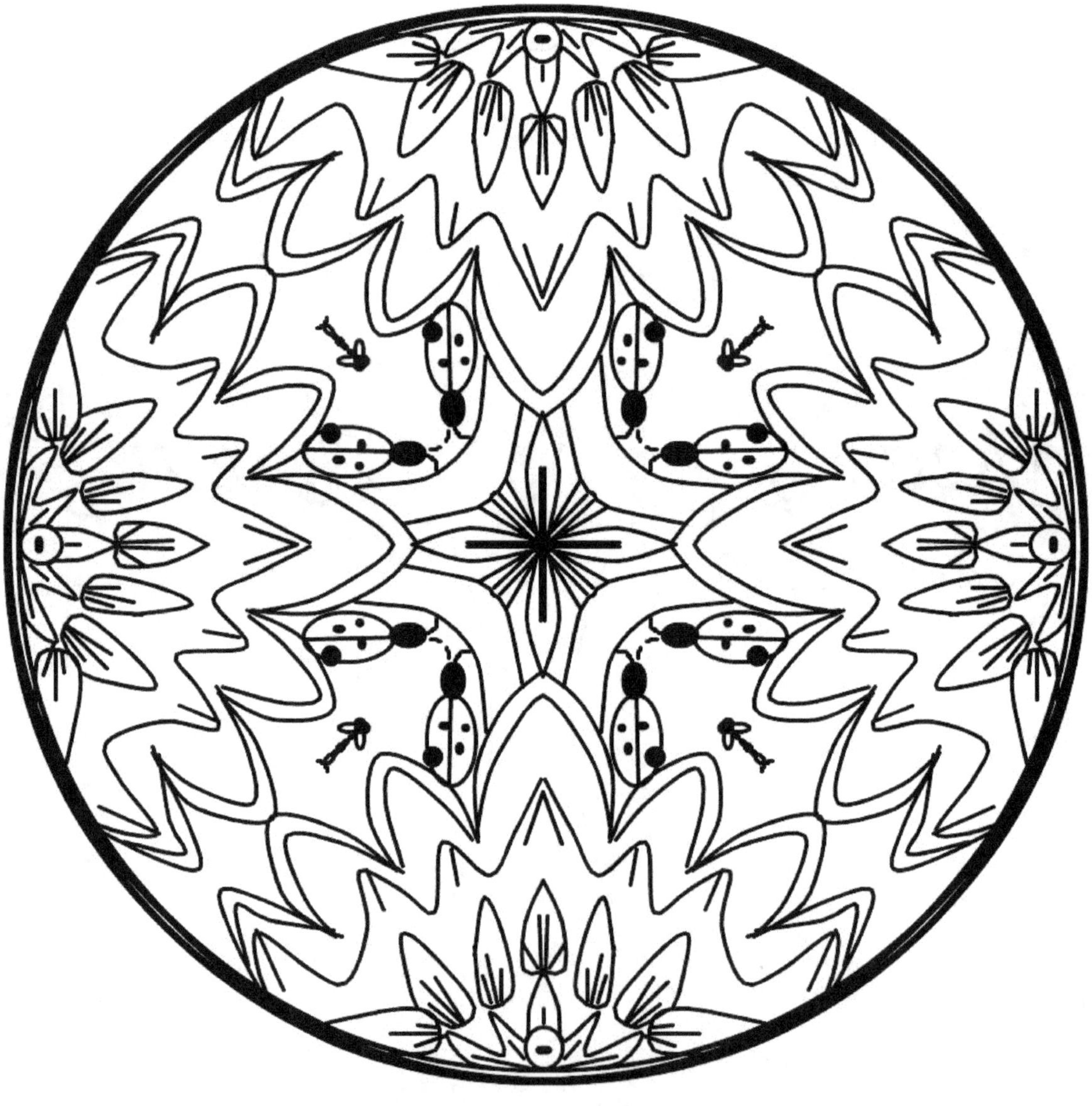

Day Seven _______

5:00 _______________________	

5:00 _____________________

6:00 _____________________

7:00 _____________________

8:00 _____________________

9:00 _____________________

10:00 _____________________

11:00 _____________________

Noon _____________________

1:00 _____________________

2:00 _____________________

3:00 _____________________

4:00 _____________________

5:00 _____________________

6:00 _____________________

7:00 _____________________

8:00 _____________________

9:00 _____________________

10:00 _____________________

11:00 _____________________

Midnight _____________________

top priorities for today

Today's victories

Where does your strength
come from?

The Training

Exercise	Set 1	Set 2	Set 3	Set 4	Set 5	notes

Time started: _____________ Time ended: _______________

Location: ____

Feelings before training:

Feelings after training

NUTRITION

Meal 1
time eaten: _________

Meal 2
time eaten: _________

Meal 3
time eaten: _________

Meal 4
time eaten: _________

Meal 5
time eaten: _________

Hydration

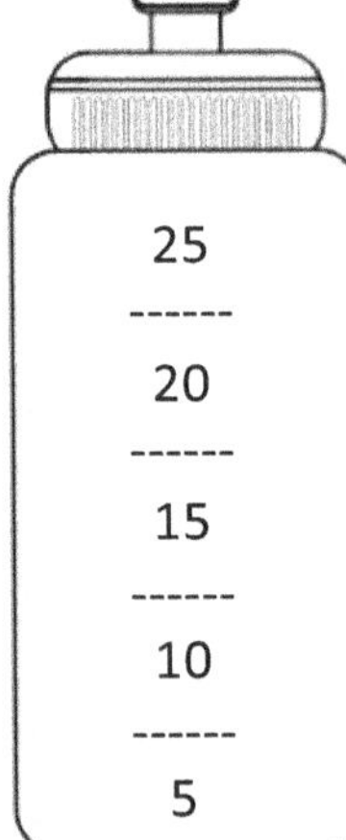 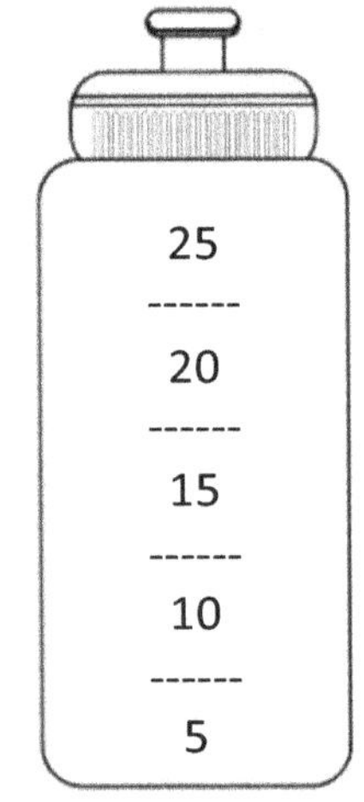 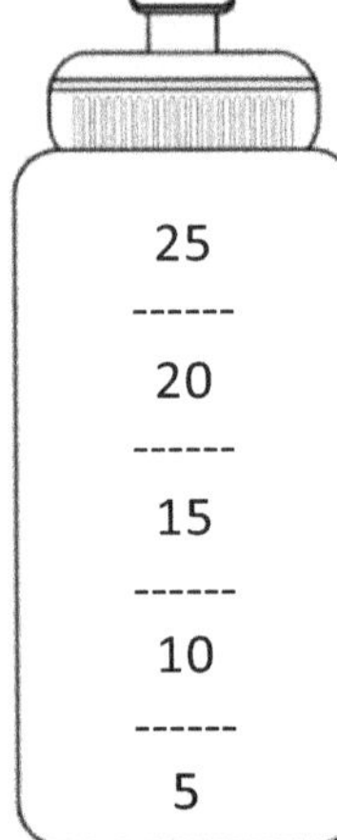 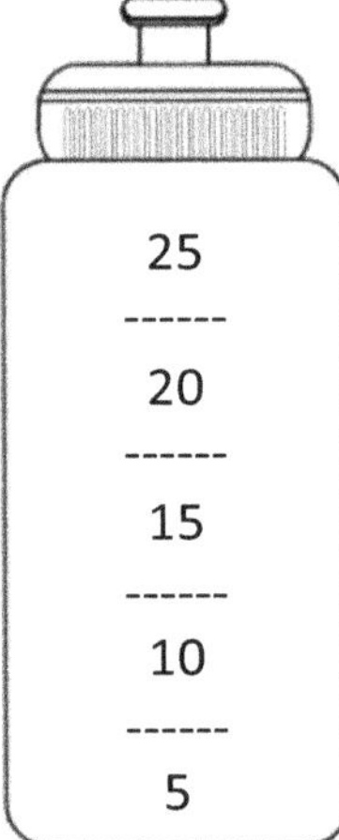 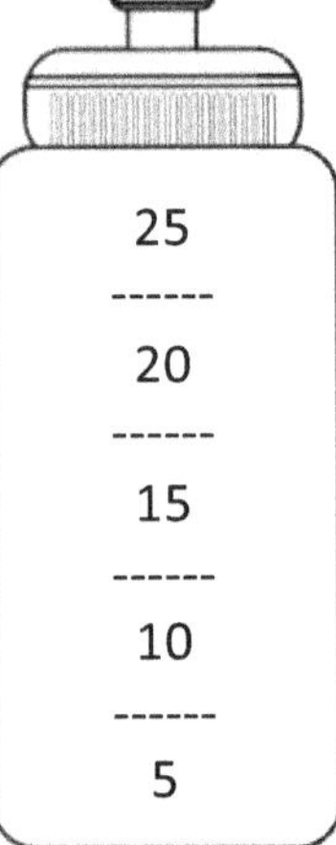

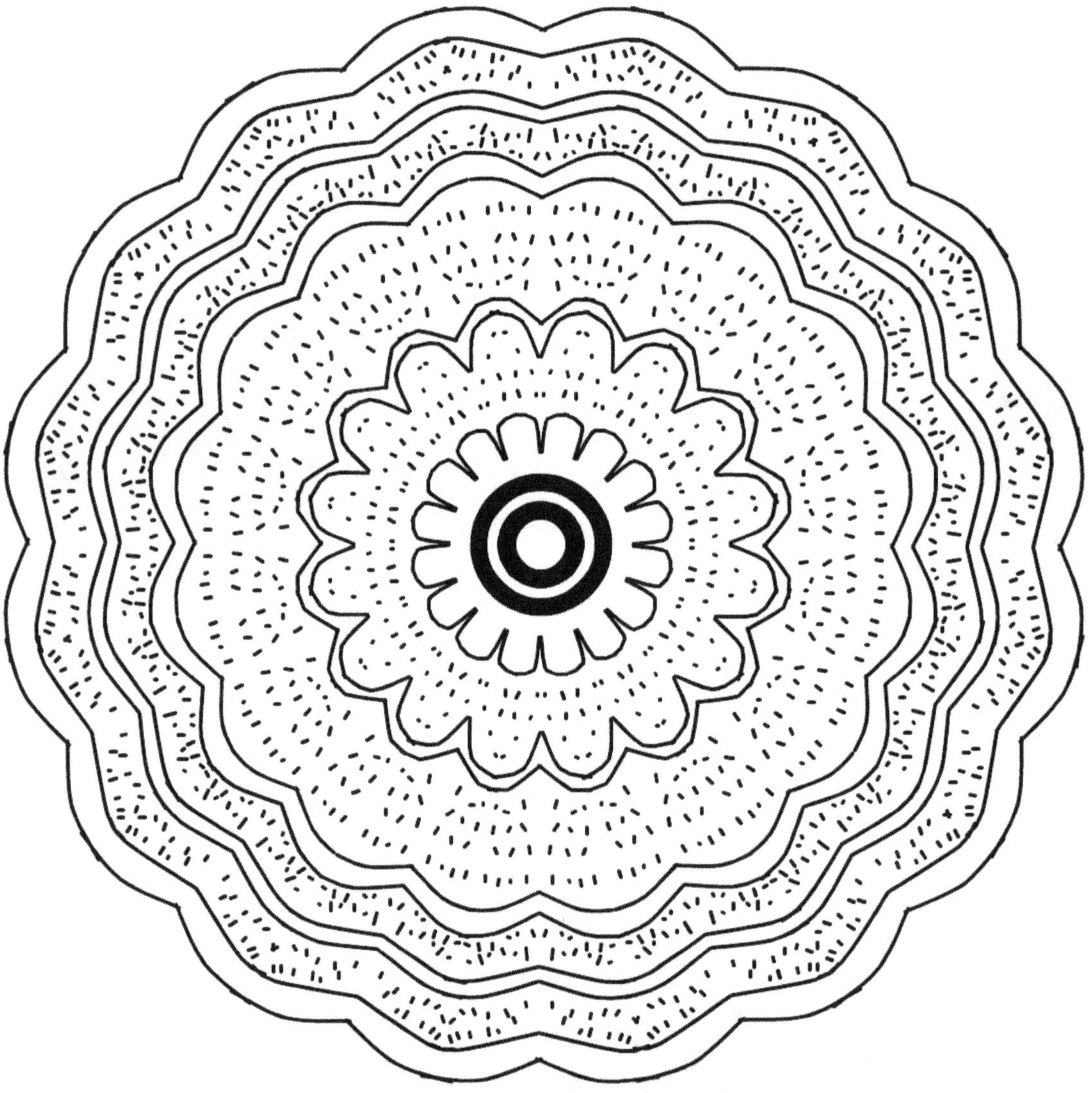

Day Eight _______

5:00 _____________	

top priorities for today 

____

____

____

____

5:00 __________________

6:00 __________________

7:00 __________________

8:00 __________________

9:00 __________________

10:00 __________________

11:00 __________________

Noon __________________

1:00 __________________

2:00 __________________

3:00 __________________

4:00 __________________

5:00 __________________

6:00 __________________

7:00 __________________

8:00 __________________

9:00 __________________

10:00 __________________

11:00 __________________

Midnight __________________

Today's victories

What motivates you to be
the best version of you?

____

____

____

____

____

____

The *Stella Society* Training

Exercise	Set 1	Set 2	Set 3	Set 4	Set 5	notes

Time started: _____________ Time ended: _____________

Location: ____

Feelings before training: 😊 😐 ☹️ 😜 😠 😕 😊 😎

Feelings after training 😊 😐 ☹️ 😜 😠 😕 😊 😎

NUTRITION

Meal 1

time eaten: _________

Meal 2

time eaten: _________

Meal 3

time eaten: _________

Meal 4

time eaten: _________

Meal 5

time eaten: _________

Hydration

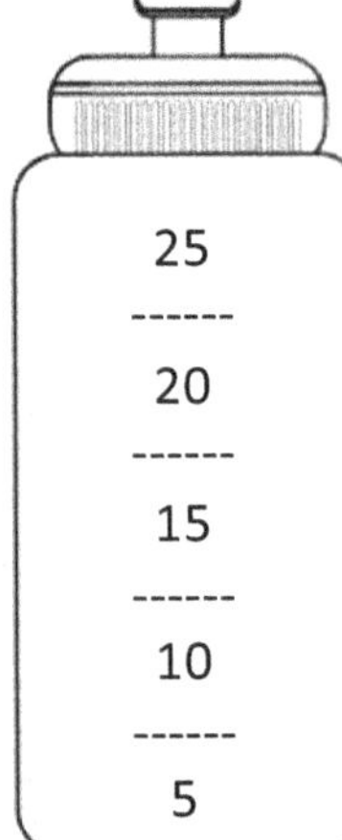
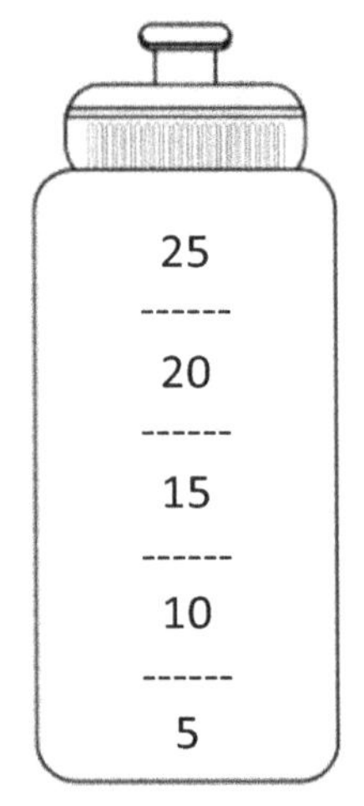
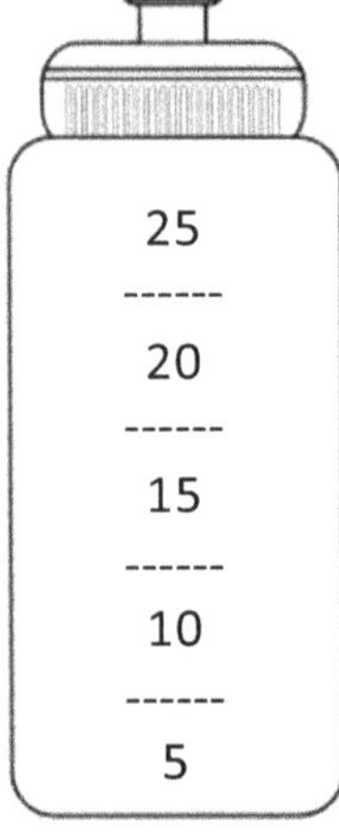
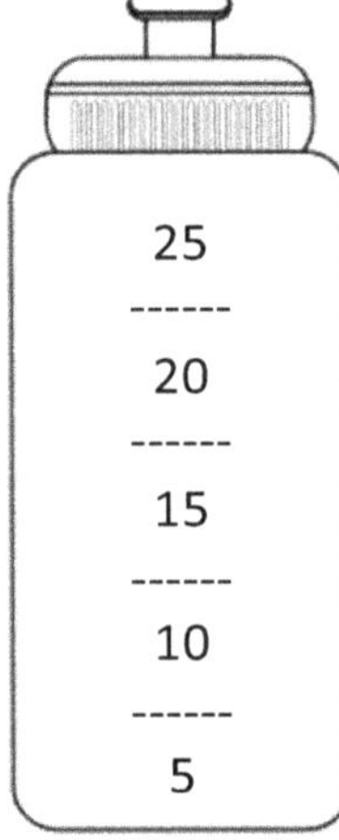
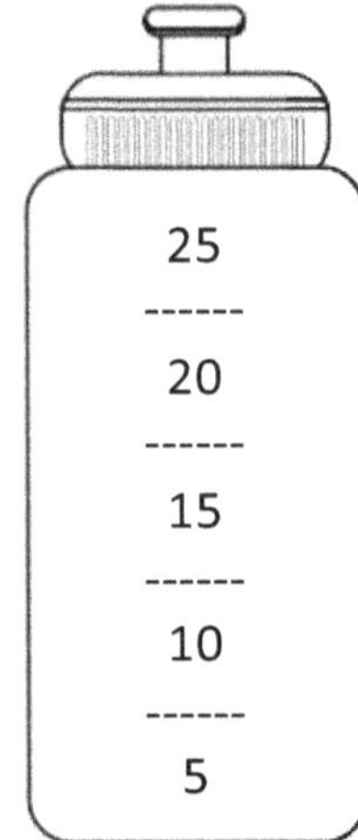

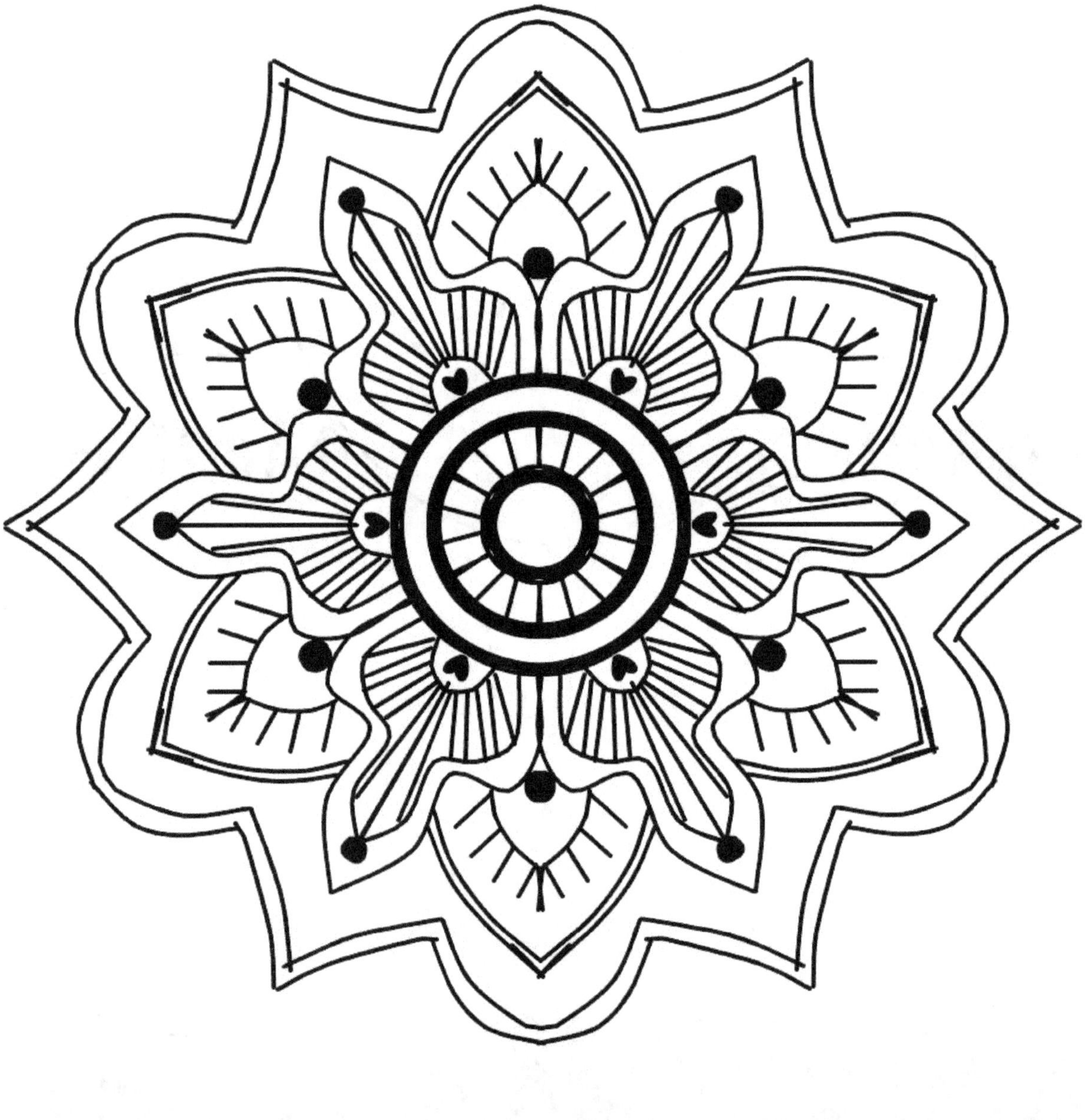

Day Nine _______

5:00 _______________________

6:00 _______________________

7:00 _______________________

8:00 _______________________

9:00 _______________________

10:00 ______________________

11:00 ______________________

Noon _______________________

1:00 _______________________

2:00 _______________________

3:00 _______________________

4:00 _______________________

5:00 _______________________

6:00 _______________________

7:00 _______________________

8:00 _______________________

9:00 _______________________

10:00 ______________________

11:00 ______________________

Midnight ___________________

top priorities for today

____
____
____
____
____

Today's victories

How will you be consistent
this week?

____
____
____
____
____
____

The ⦿ Stella Society Training

Exercise	Set 1	Set 2	Set 3	Set 4	Set 5	notes

Time started: _____________ Time ended: ______________

Location: ____

Feelings before training: 🙂 😐 🙁 😜 😠 😕 😊 😎

Feelings after training 🙂 😐 🙁 😜 😠 😕 😊 😎

NUTRITION

Meal 1

time eaten: _________

Meal 2

time eaten: _________

Meal 3

time eaten: _________

Meal 4

time eaten: _________

Meal 5

time eaten: _________

Hydration

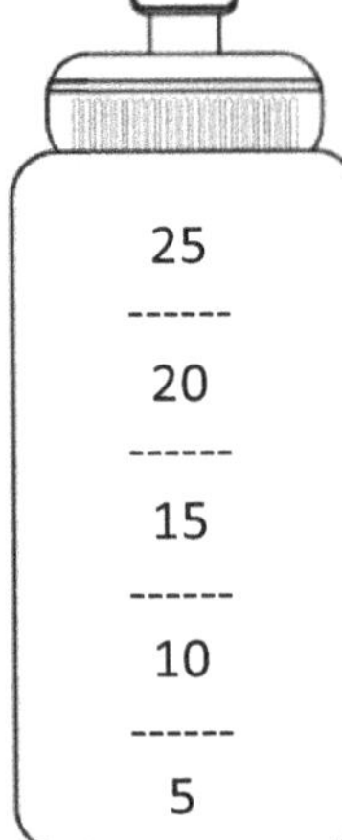

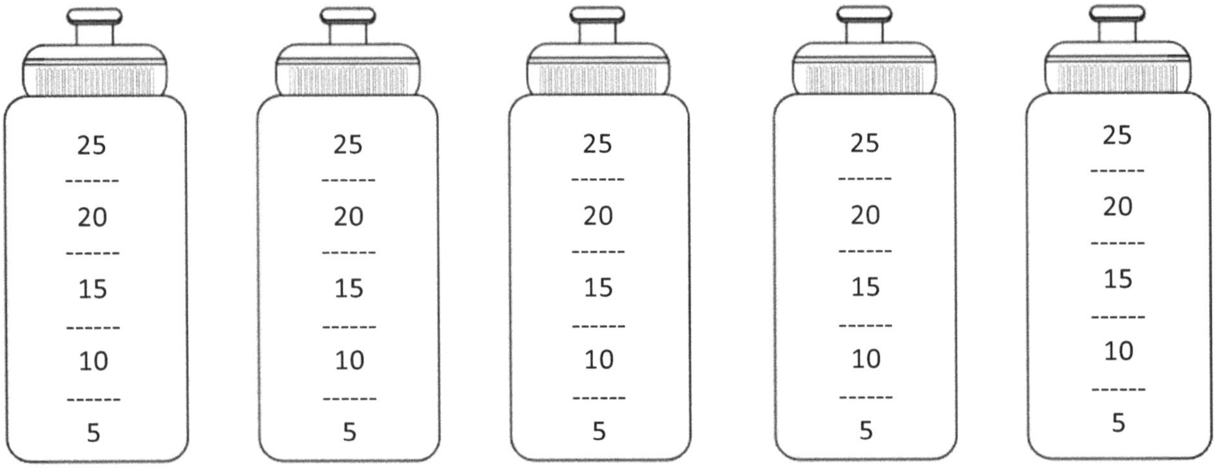

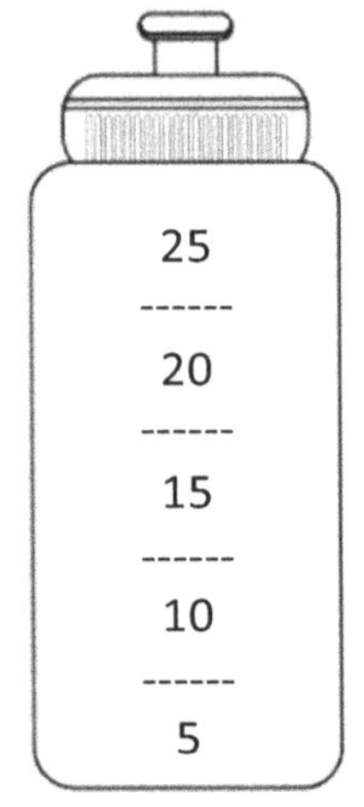

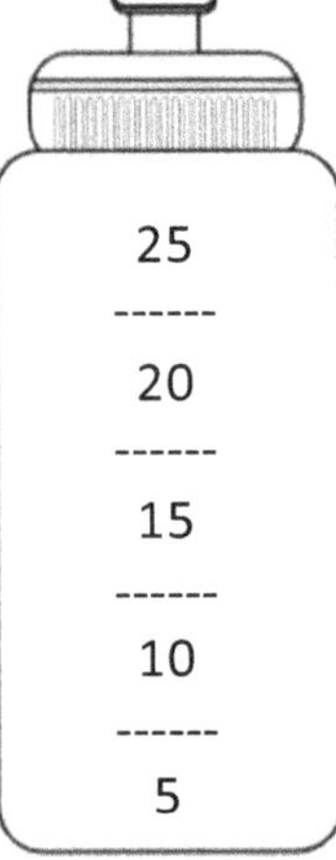

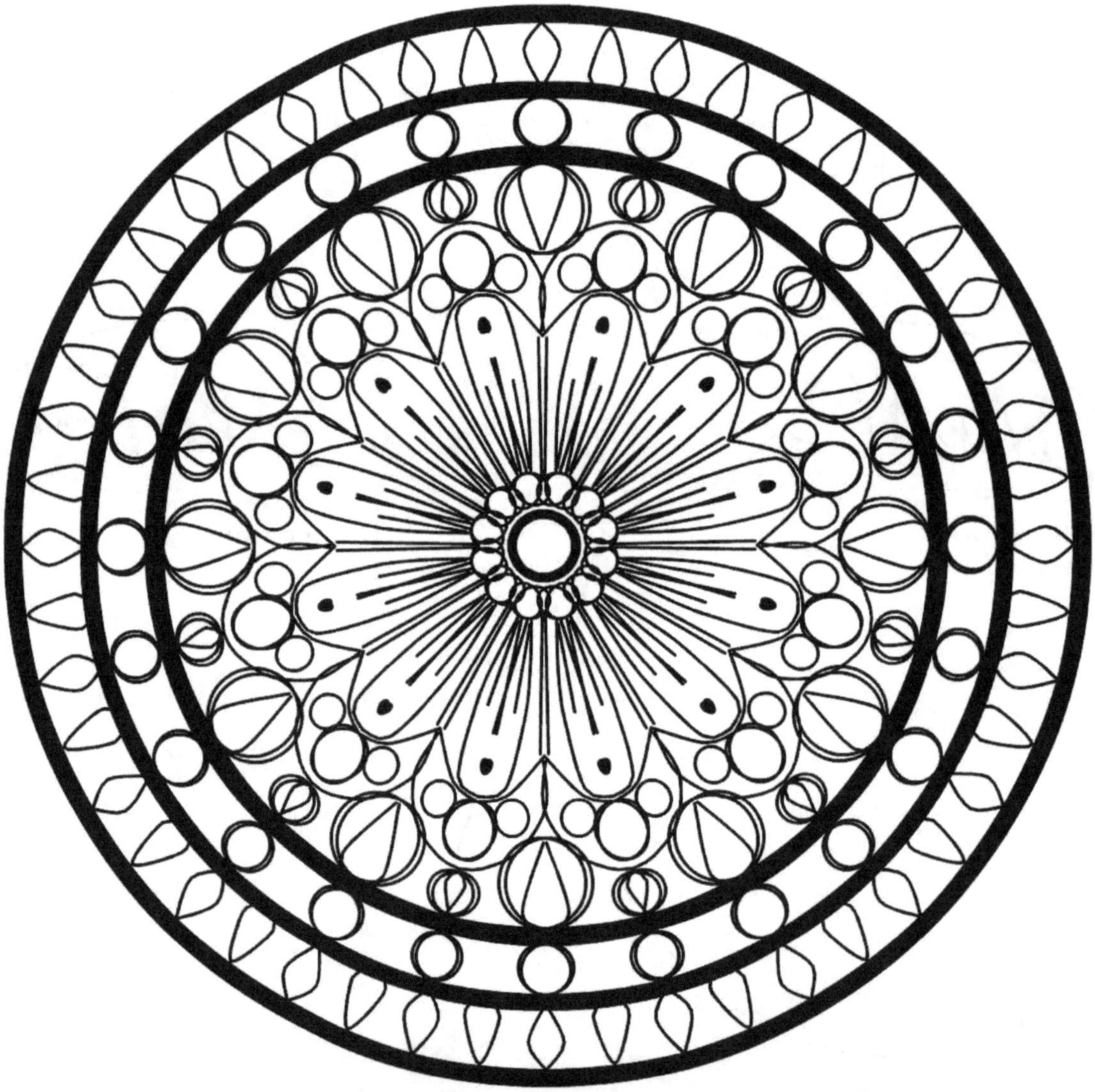

Day Ten _______

<table>
<tr><td>

5:00 _______________________

6:00 _______________________

7:00 _______________________

8:00 _______________________

9:00 _______________________

10:00 ______________________

11:00 ______________________

Noon _______________________

1:00 _______________________

2:00 _______________________

3:00 _______________________

4:00 _______________________

5:00 _______________________

6:00 _______________________

7:00 _______________________

8:00 _______________________

9:00 _______________________

10:00 ______________________

11:00 ______________________

Midnight ___________________

</td><td>

top priorities for today 🎯

____

____

____

____

Today's victories 🏆

List 5 ways you are loving.

____

____

____

____

____

____

</td></tr>
</table>

The Training

Exercise	Set 1	Set 2	Set 3	Set 4	Set 5	notes

Time started: _____________   Time ended: _____________

Location: ____

Feelings before training:

Feelings after training

NUTRITION

Meal 1
time eaten: _________

Meal 2
time eaten: _________

Meal 3
time eaten: _________

Meal 4
time eaten: _________

Meal 5
time eaten: _________

Hydration

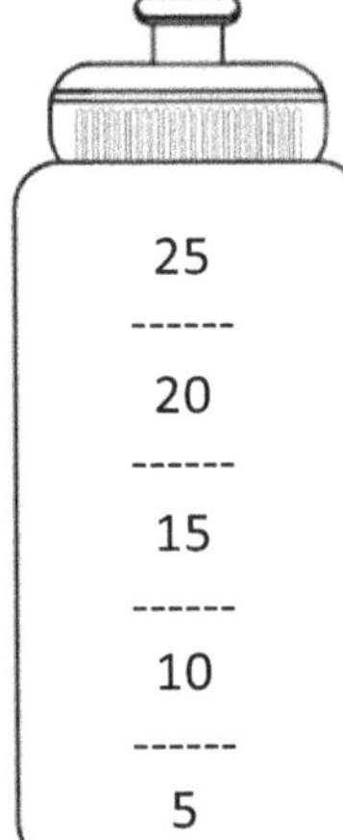

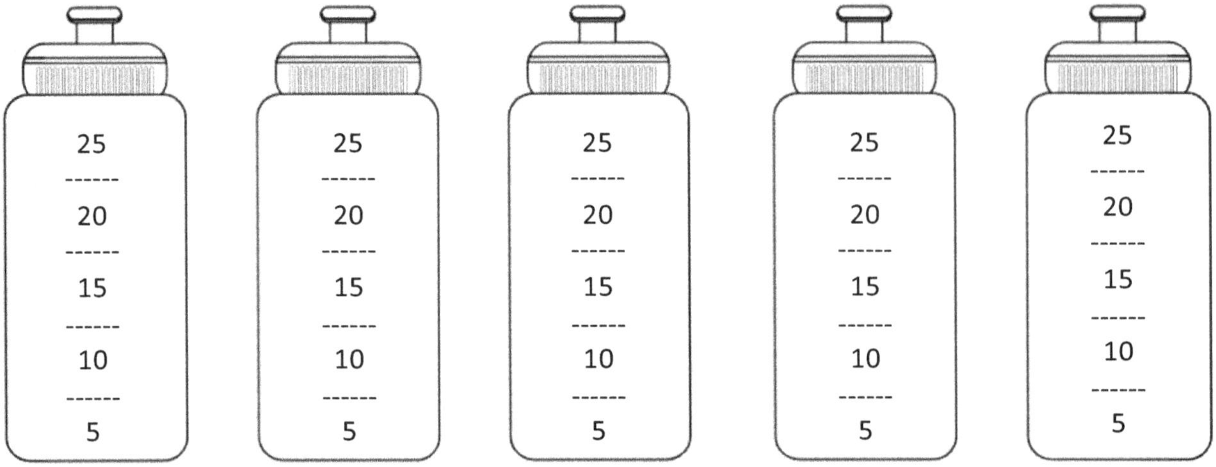

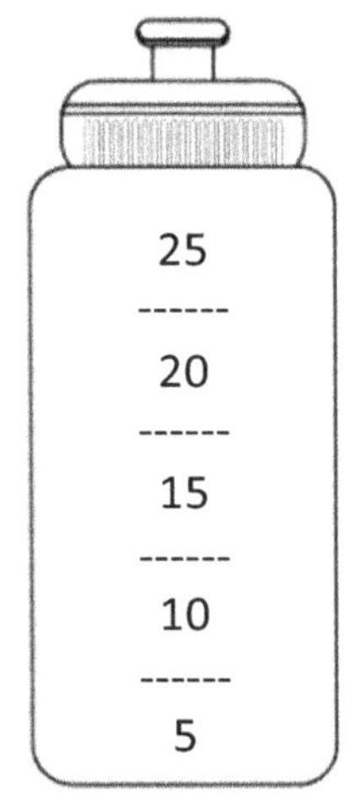

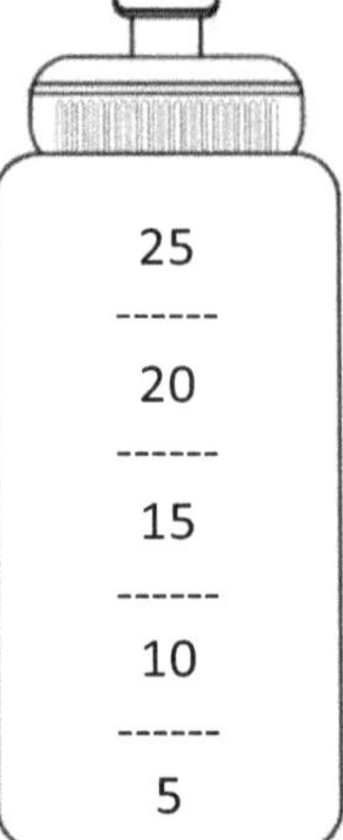

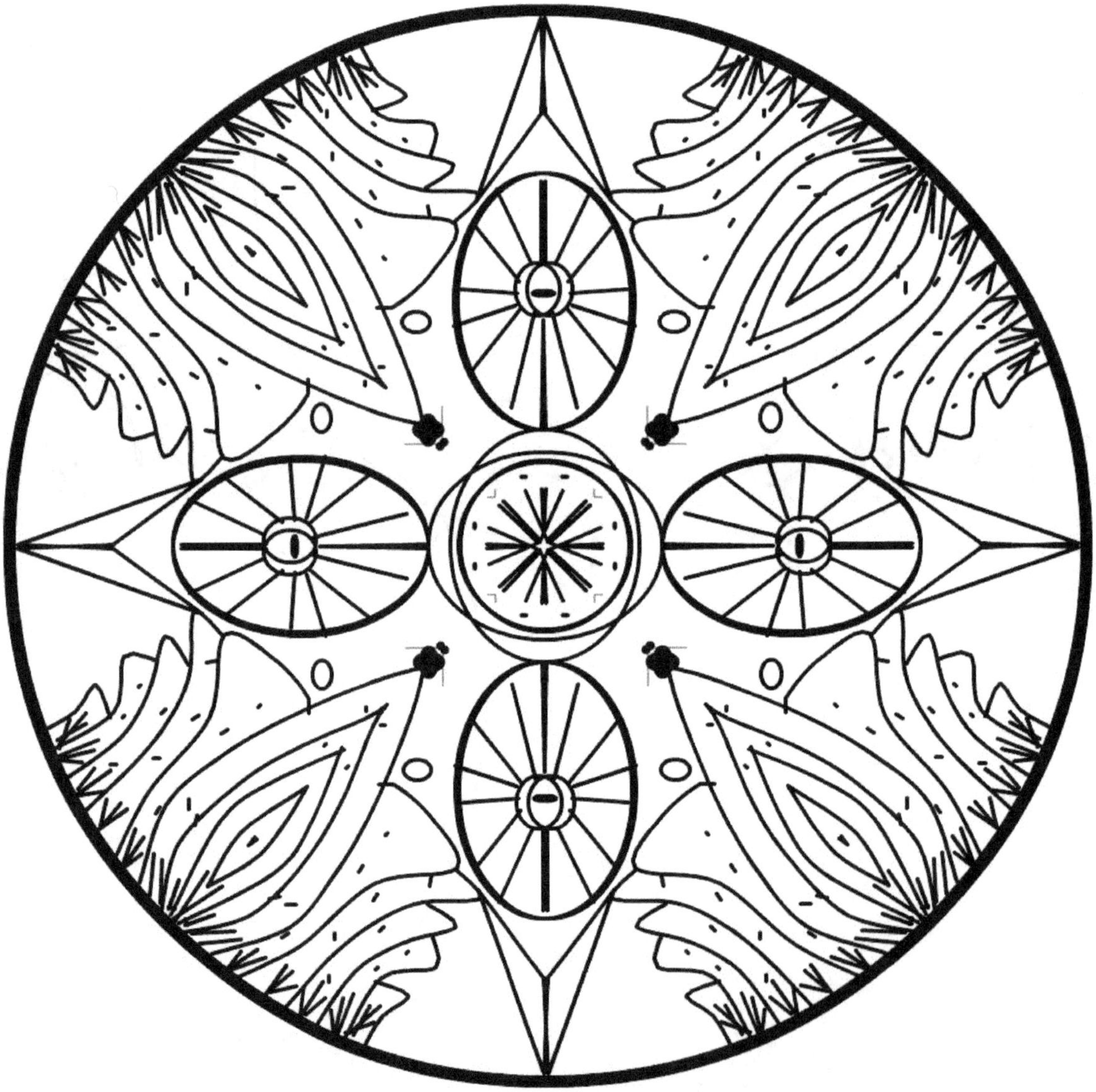

Measurements

P R O G R E S S

DATE: ____________

Weight: _______

Neck _______

Shoulders _______

Chest _______

Bicep / upper arm left _________ right _______

Forearm left _________ right _______

Waist _______

Hips _______

Thighs left _________ right _____

Calf left _________ right _______

C H E C K

The Struggle You Are In Today, Is Developing The Strength You Need for Tomorrow.

Day Eleven _______

5:00 _______________________

6:00 _______________________

7:00 _______________________

8:00 _______________________

9:00 _______________________

10:00 ______________________

11:00 ______________________

Noon _______________________

1:00 _______________________

2:00 _______________________

3:00 _______________________

4:00 _______________________

5:00 _______________________

6:00 _______________________

7:00 _______________________

8:00 _______________________

9:00 _______________________

10:00 ______________________

11:00 ______________________

Midnight ___________________

Today's victories

Give out as many hugs as you can today. How many did you give?

The Training

Exercise	Set 1	Set 2	Set 3	Set 4	Set 5	notes

Time started: _______________   Time ended: _________________

Location: ____

Feelings before training:       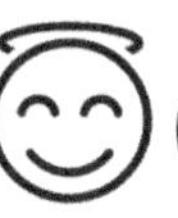 

Feelings after training

NUTRITION

Meal 1
time eaten: _________

Meal 2
time eaten: _________

Meal 3
time eaten: _________

Meal 4
time eaten: _________

Meal 5
time eaten: _________

Hydration

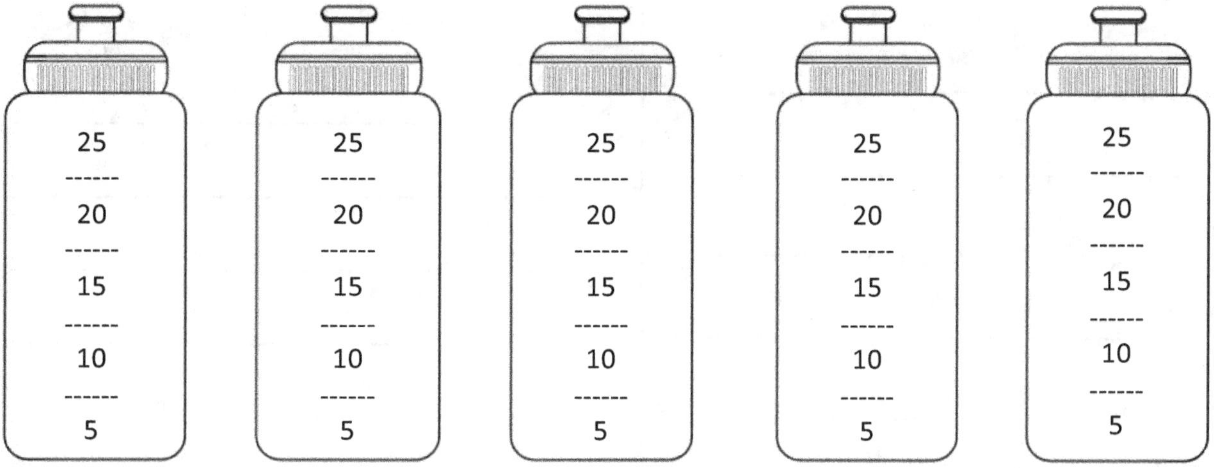

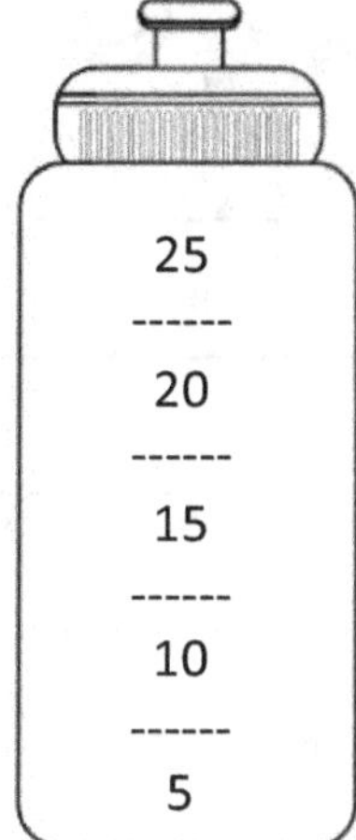
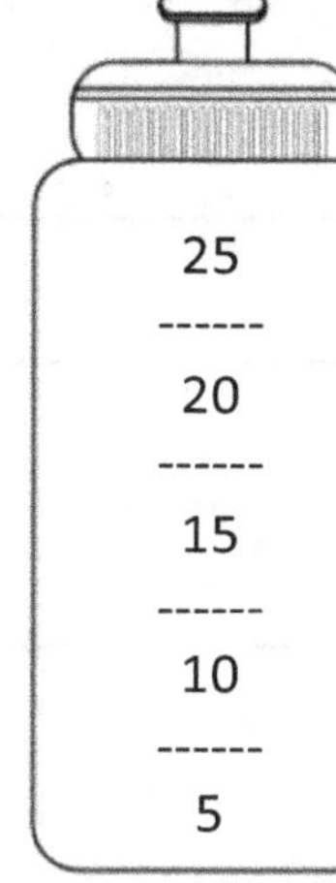

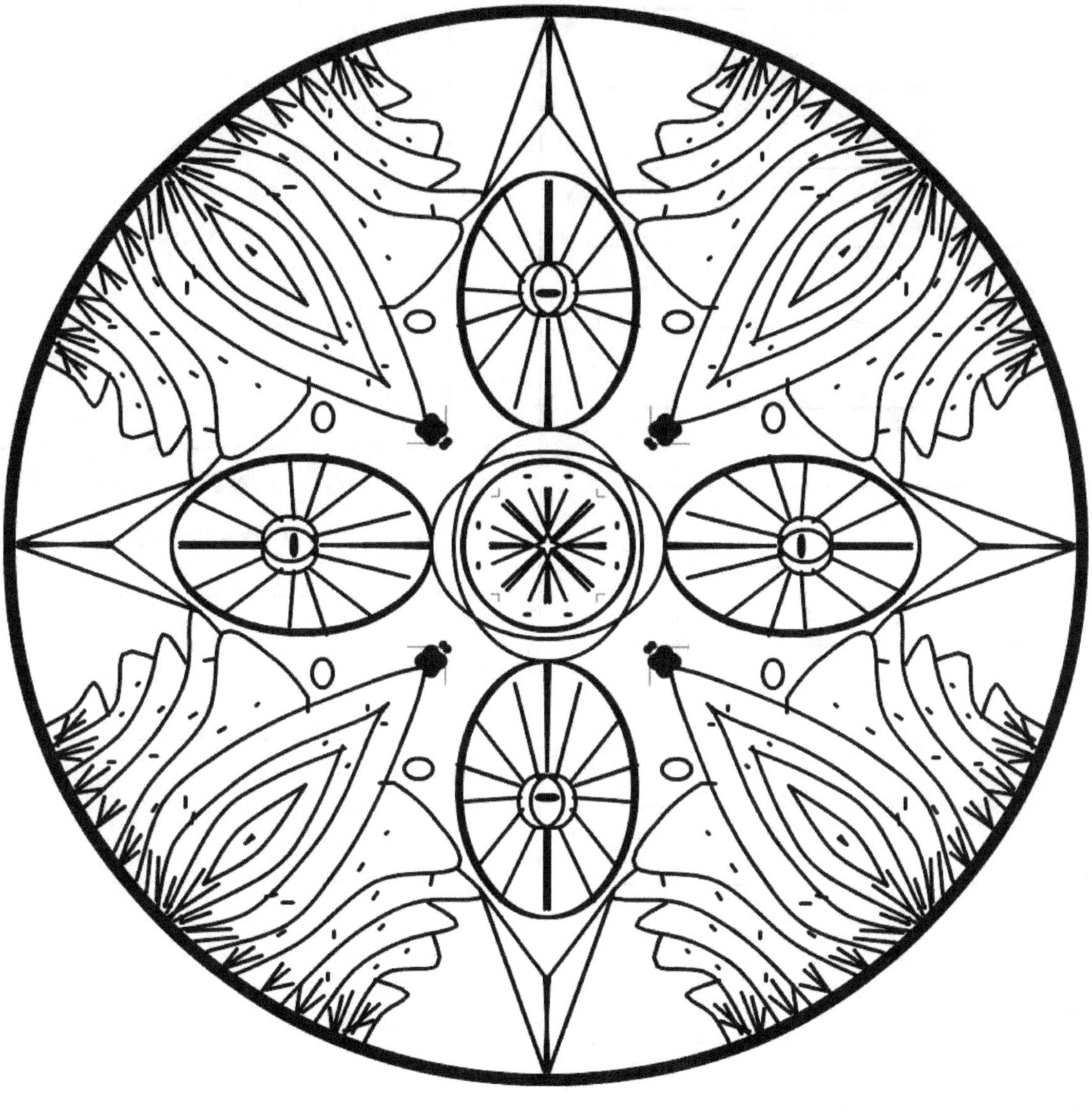

Day Twelve _______

5:00 _______________________

6:00 _______________________

7:00 _______________________

8:00 _______________________

9:00 _______________________

10:00 _______________________

11:00 _______________________

Noon _______________________

1:00 _______________________

2:00 _______________________

3:00 _______________________

4:00 _______________________

5:00 _______________________

6:00 _______________________

7:00 _______________________

8:00 _______________________

9:00 _______________________

10:00 _______________________

11:00 _______________________

Midnight _______________________

top priorities for today

____

____

____

____

____

Today's victories

List 4 ways you show compassion.

____

____

____

____

____

The Training

Exercise	Set 1	Set 2	Set 3	Set 4	Set 5	notes

Time started: ______________ Time ended: ________________

Location: ____

Feelings before training: 

Feelings after training

NUTRITION

Meal 1

time eaten: _________

Meal 2

time eaten: _________

Meal 3

time eaten: _________

Meal 4

time eaten: _________

Meal 5

time eaten: _________

Hydration

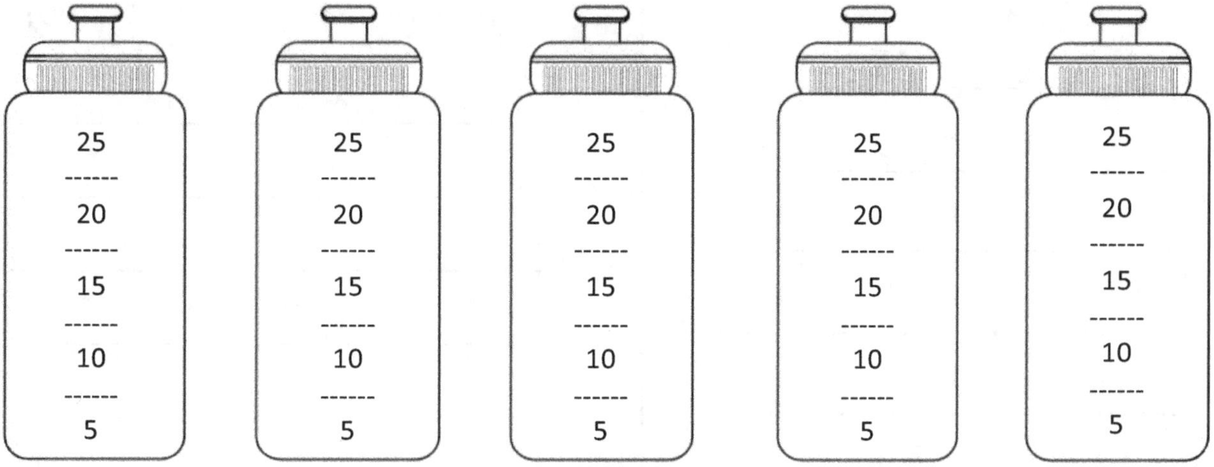

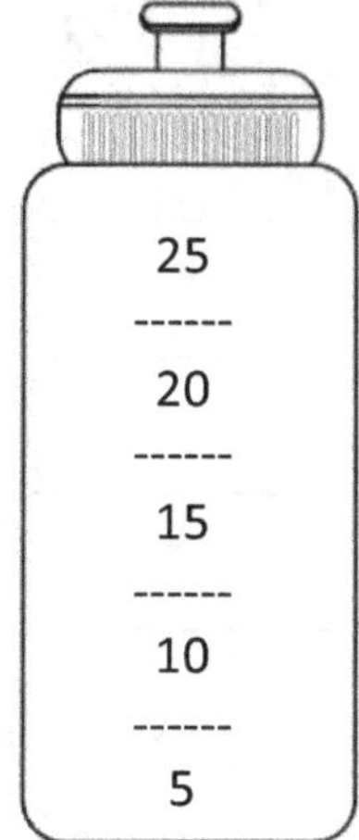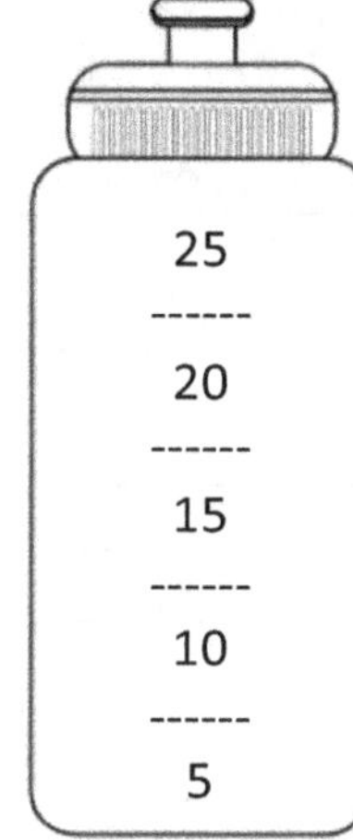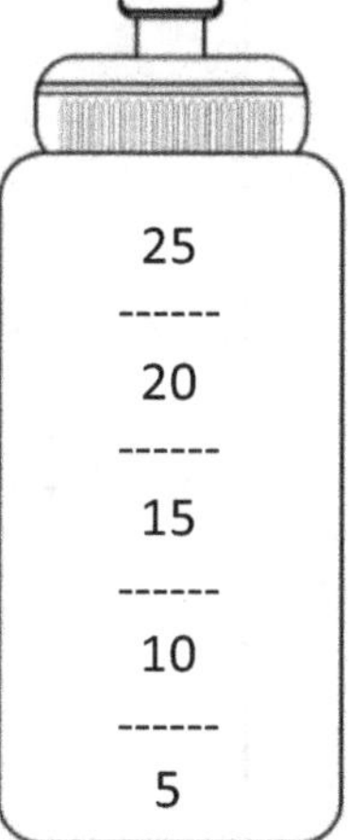

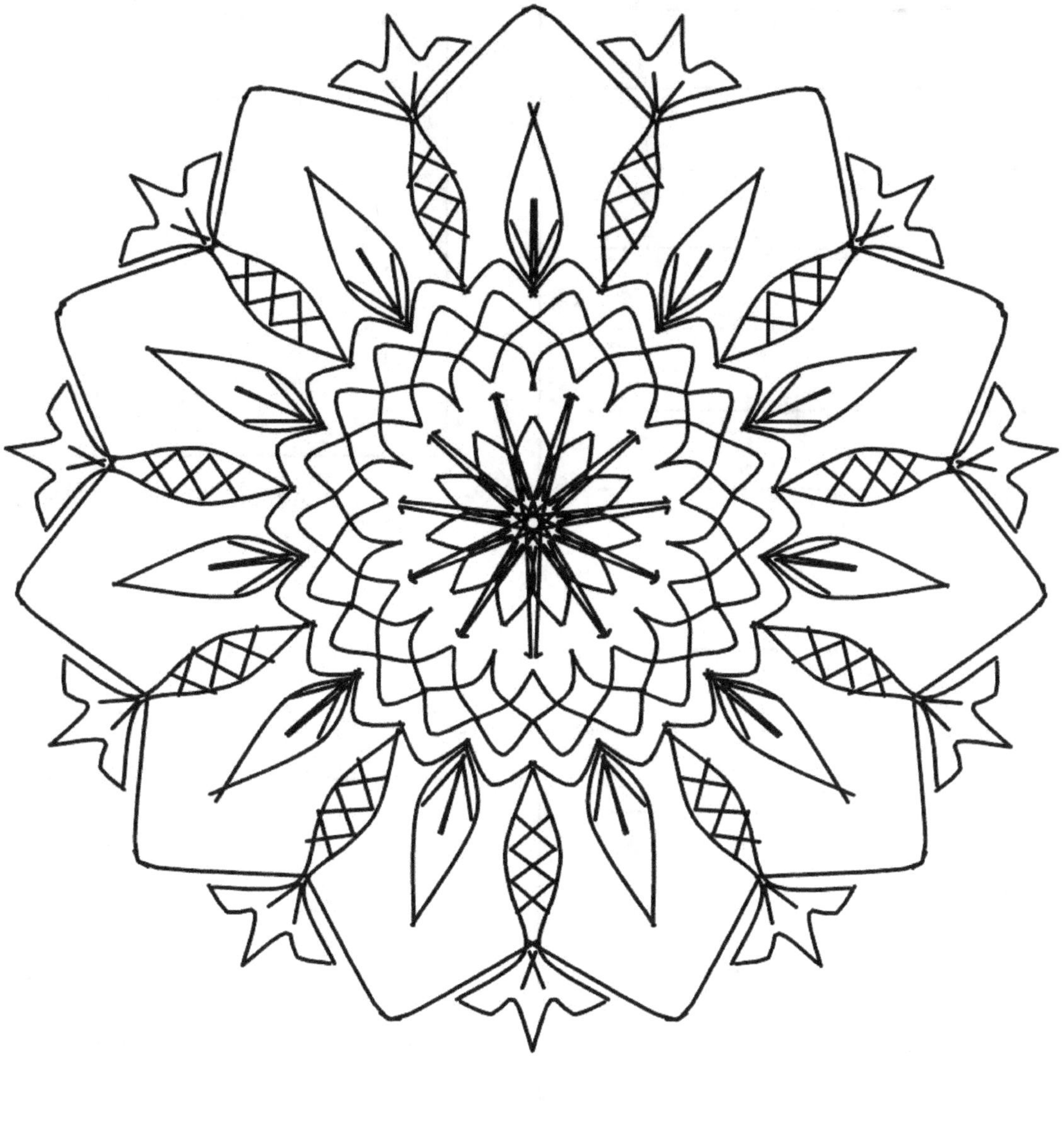

Day Thirteen _______

5:00 __________	

5:00 ____________________

6:00 ____________________

7:00 ____________________

8:00 ____________________

9:00 ____________________

10:00 ____________________

11:00 ____________________

Noon ____________________

1:00 ____________________

2:00 ____________________

3:00 ____________________

4:00 ____________________

5:00 ____________________

6:00 ____________________

7:00 ____________________

8:00 ____________________

9:00 ____________________

10:00 ____________________

11:00 ____________________

Midnight ____________________

top priorities for today

____

____

____

____

Today's victories 🏆

Who needs roses from your
garden and why?

____

____

____

____

____

m# The   Stella Society   Training

Exercise	Set 1	Set 2	Set 3	Set 4	Set 5	notes

Time started: _______________ Time ended: _______________

Location: ____

Feelings before training: 🙂 😐 🙁 😜 😠 😕 😊 😎

Feelings after training 🙂 😐 🙁 😜 😠 😕 😊 😎

NUTRITION

Meal 1

time eaten: _________

Meal 2

time eaten: _________

Meal 3

time eaten: _________

Meal 4

time eaten: _________

Meal 5

time eaten: _________

Hydration

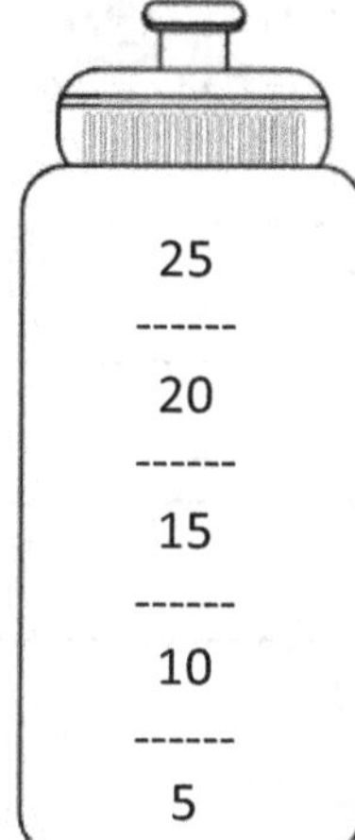 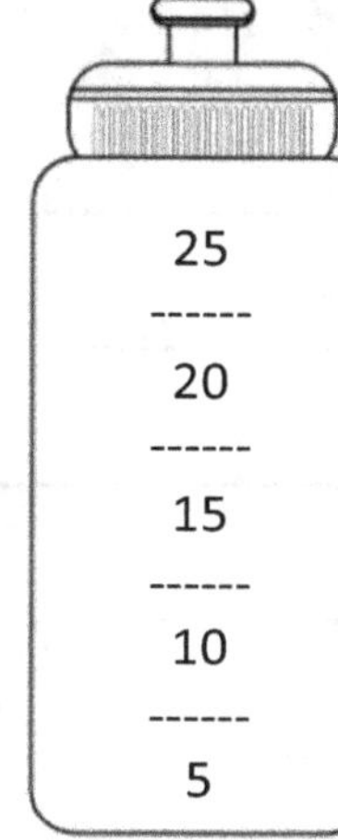 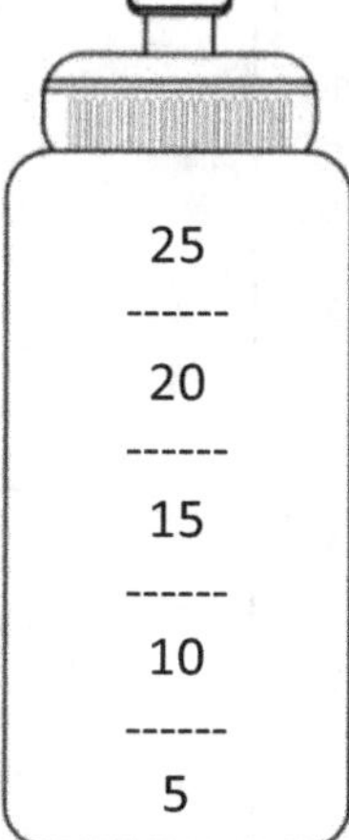

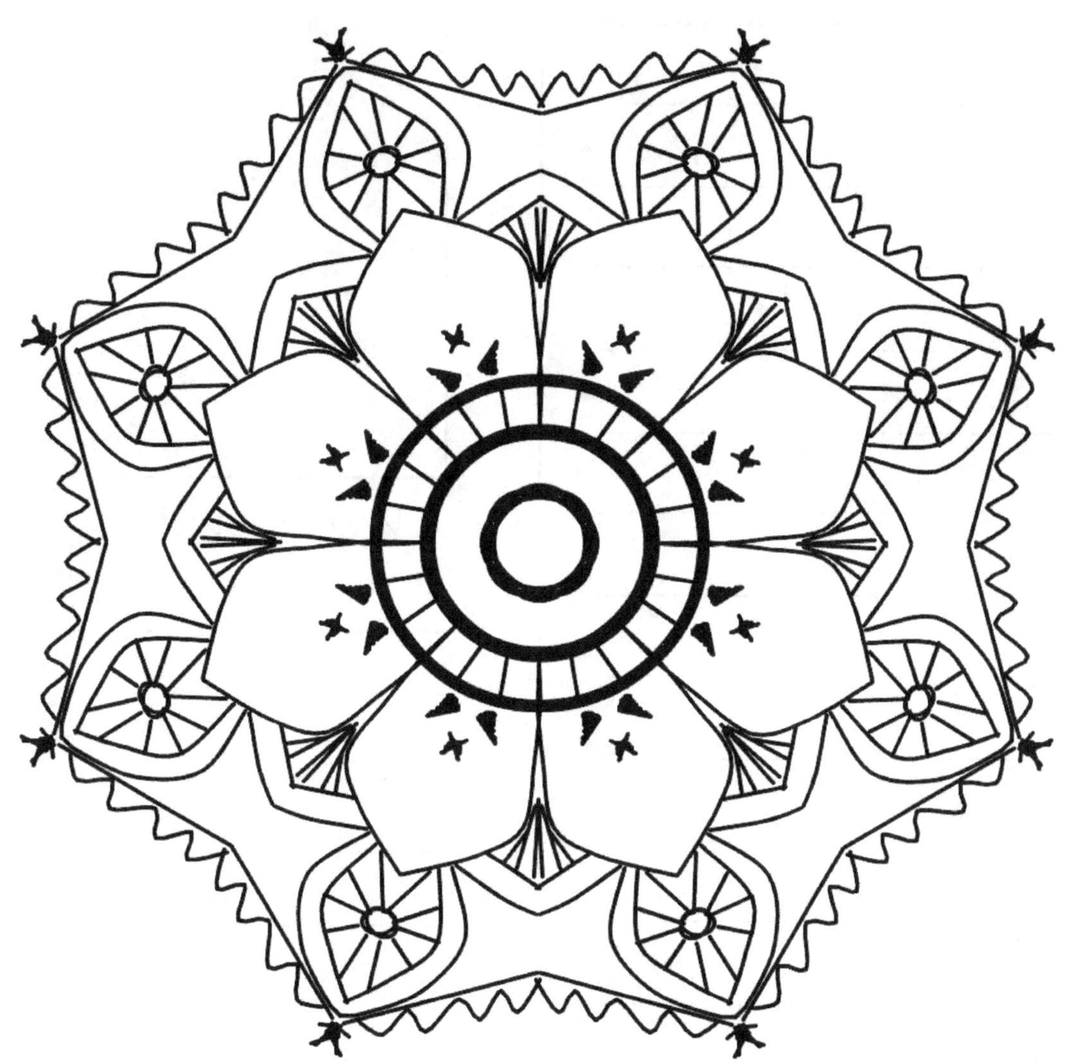

Day Fourteen _______

5:00 _______________________

6:00 _______________________

7:00 _______________________

8:00 _______________________

9:00 _______________________

10:00 ______________________

11:00 ______________________

Noon _______________________

1:00 _______________________

2:00 _______________________

3:00 _______________________

4:00 _______________________

5:00 _______________________

6:00 _______________________

7:00 _______________________

8:00 _______________________

9:00 _______________________

10:00 ______________________

11:00 ______________________

Midnight ____________________

____

____

____

____

____

Today's victories

What should you forgive your self for?

____

____

____

____

____

The Training

Exercise	Set 1	Set 2	Set 3	Set 4	Set 5	notes

Time started: _____________ Time ended: _____________

Location: ____

Feelings before training:       

Feelings after training

NUTRITION

Meal 1

time eaten: _________

Meal 2

time eaten: _________

Meal 3

time eaten: _________

Meal 4

time eaten: _________

Meal 5

time eaten: _________

Hydration

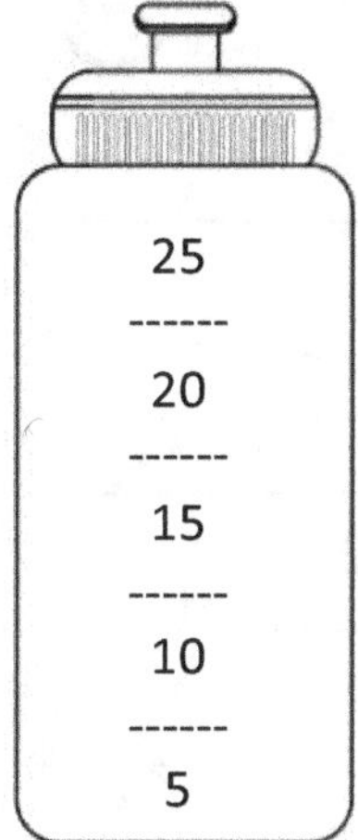

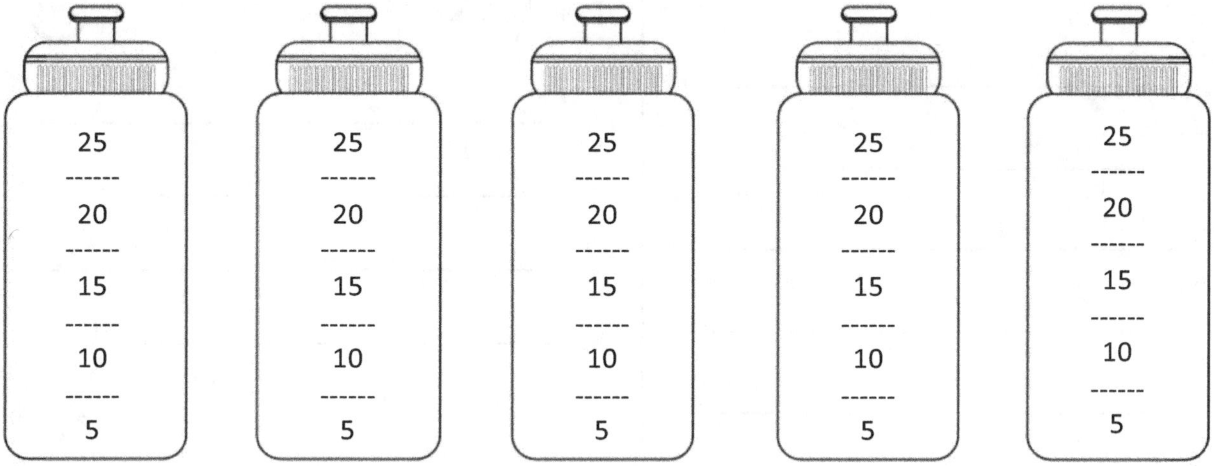

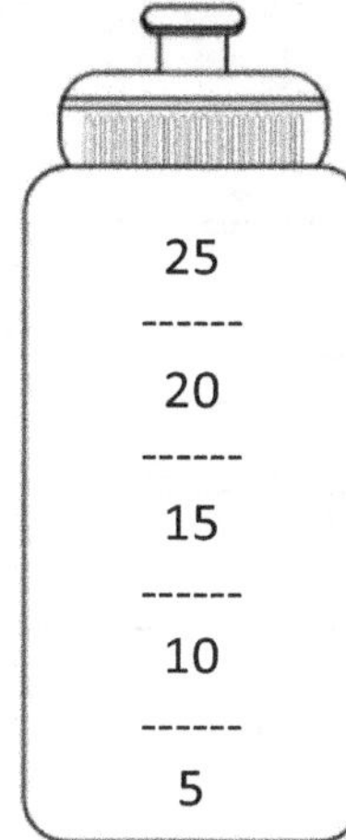

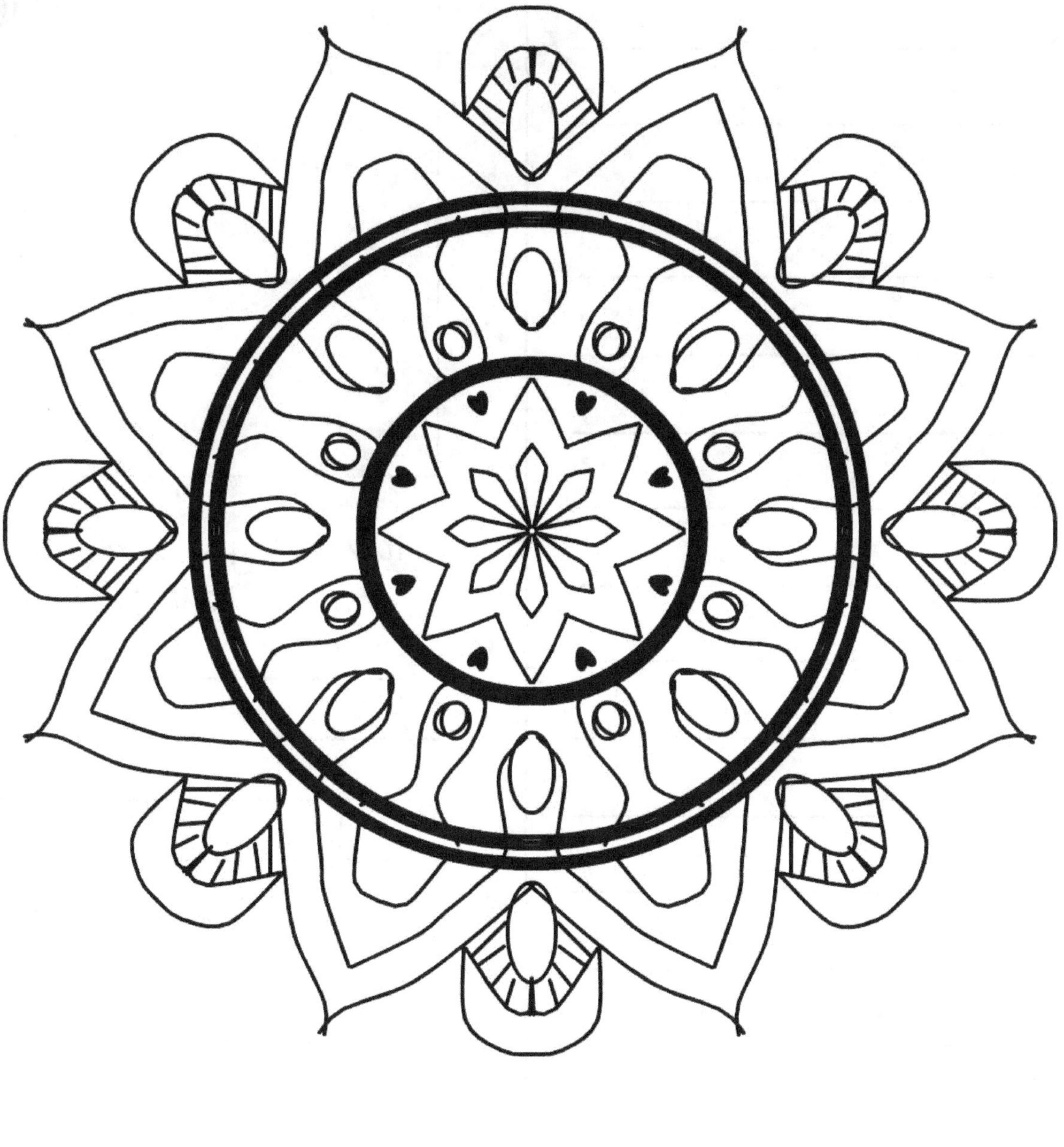

Day Fifteen _______

5:00 _______________________

6:00 _______________________

7:00 _______________________

8:00 _______________________

9:00 _______________________

10:00 ______________________

11:00 ______________________

Noon _______________________

1:00 _______________________

2:00 _______________________

3:00 _______________________

4:00 _______________________

5:00 _______________________

6:00 _______________________

7:00 _______________________

8:00 _______________________

9:00 _______________________

10:00 ______________________

11:00 ______________________

Midnight _____________

top priorities for today 🎯

____

____

____

____

____

Today's victories 🏆

How will you be remarkable today?

____

____

____

____

____

____

The Training

Exercise	Set 1	Set 2	Set 3	Set 4	Set 5	notes

Time started: _____________ Time ended: _______________

Location: ____

Feelings before training:        

Feelings after training

NUTRITION

Meal 1

time eaten: _________

Meal 2

time eaten: _________

Meal 3

time eaten: _________

Meal 4

time eaten: _________

Meal 5

time eaten: _________

Hydration

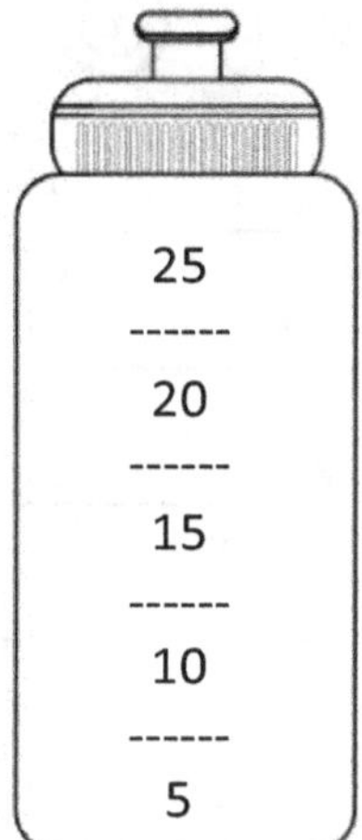

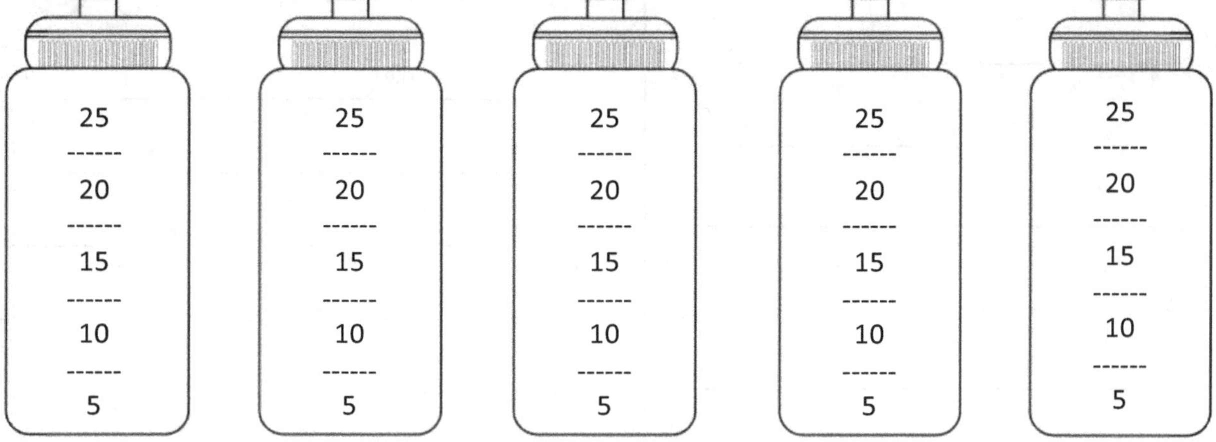

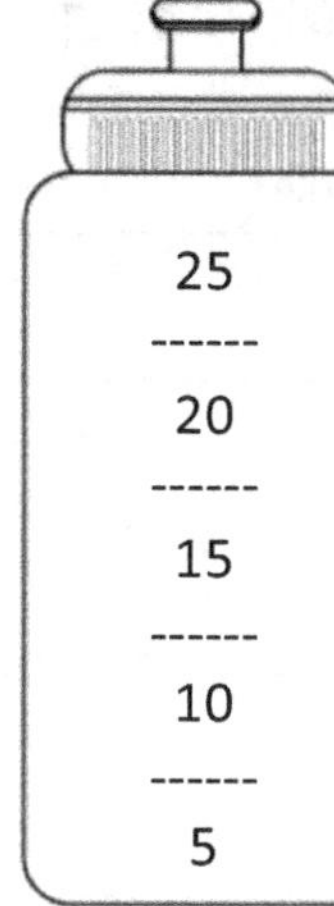

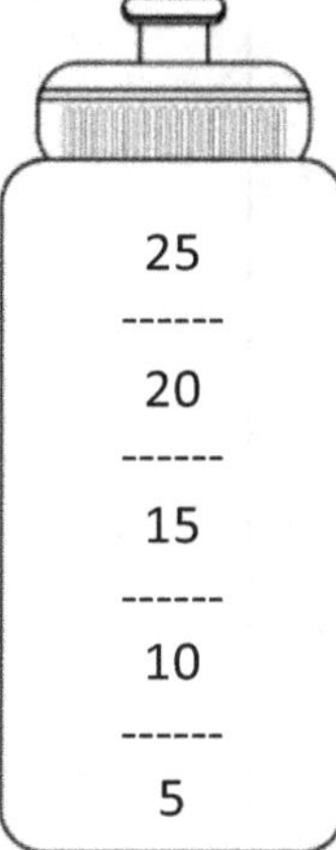

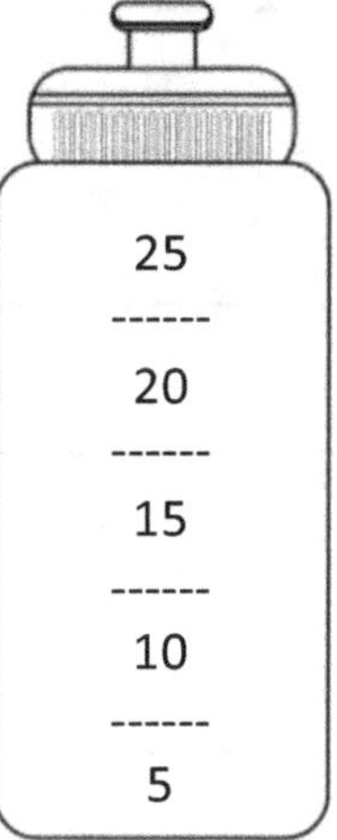

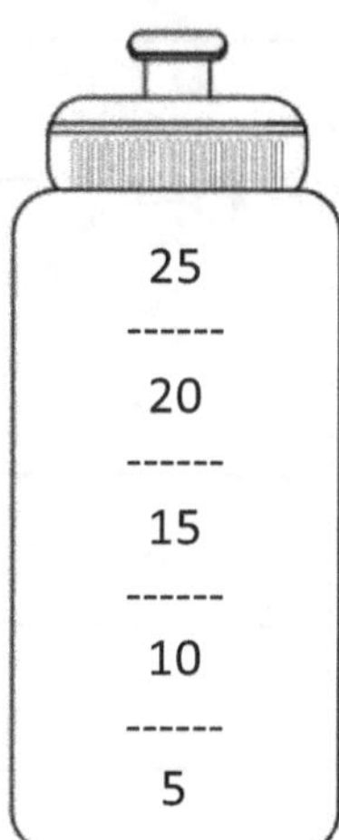

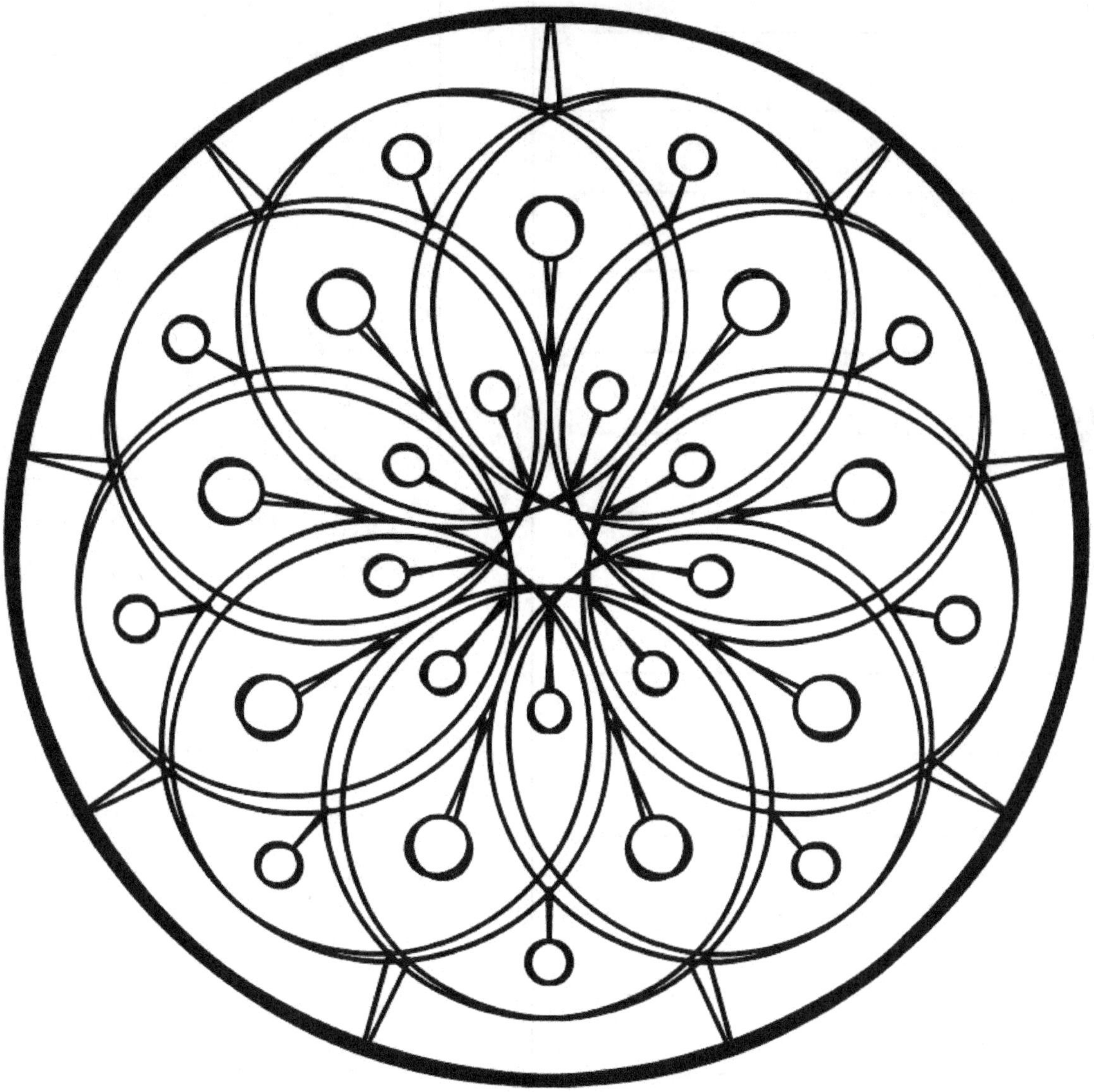

Day Sixteen _______

5:00 _______________________

6:00 _______________________

7:00 _______________________

8:00 _______________________

9:00 _______________________

10:00 ______________________

11:00 ______________________

Noon _______________________

1:00 _______________________

2:00 _______________________

3:00 _______________________

4:00 _______________________

5:00 _______________________

6:00 _______________________

7:00 _______________________

8:00 _______________________

9:00 _______________________

10:00 ______________________

11:00 ______________________

Midnight ___________________

____

____

____

____

Today's victories

Watch the sunset and list 5
places you want to see it happen?

____

____

____

____

____

____

____

The Training

Exercise	Set 1	Set 2	Set 3	Set 4	Set 5	notes

Time started: _____________   Time ended: _______________

Location: ____

Feelings before training:

Feelings after training

NUTRITION

Meal 1
time eaten: _________

Meal 2
time eaten: _________

Meal 3
time eaten: _________

Meal 4
time eaten: _________

Meal 5
time eaten: _________

Hydration

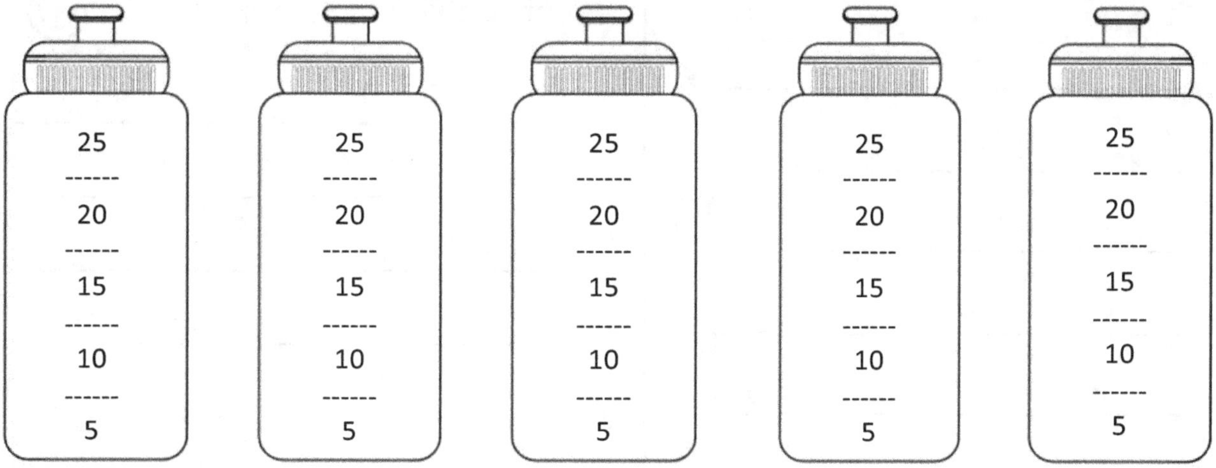

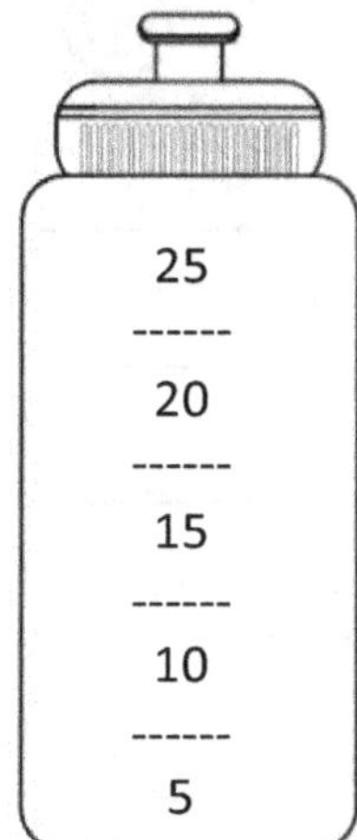
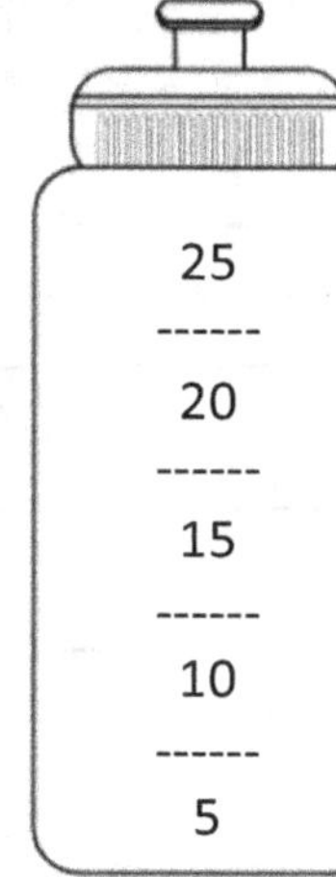
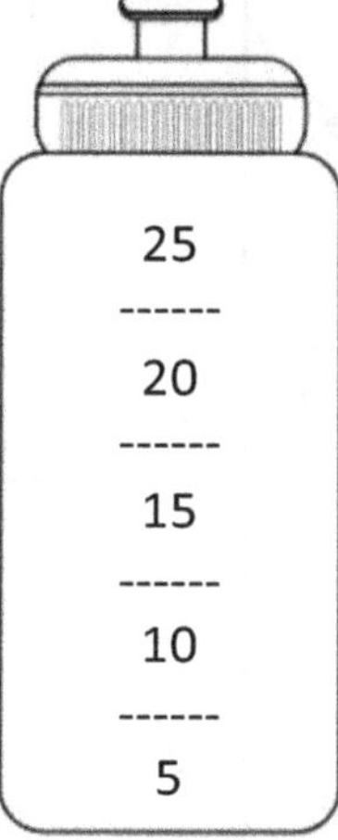
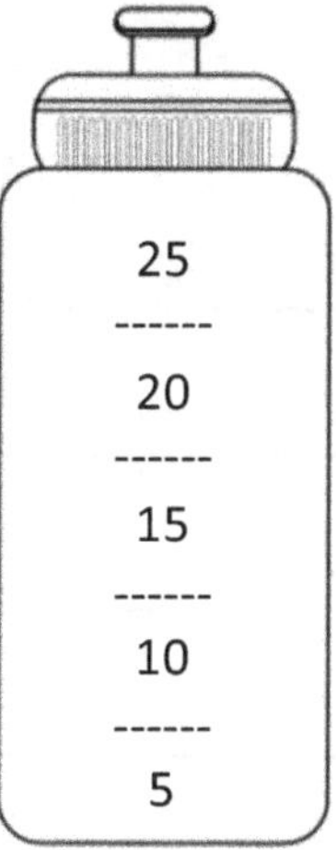

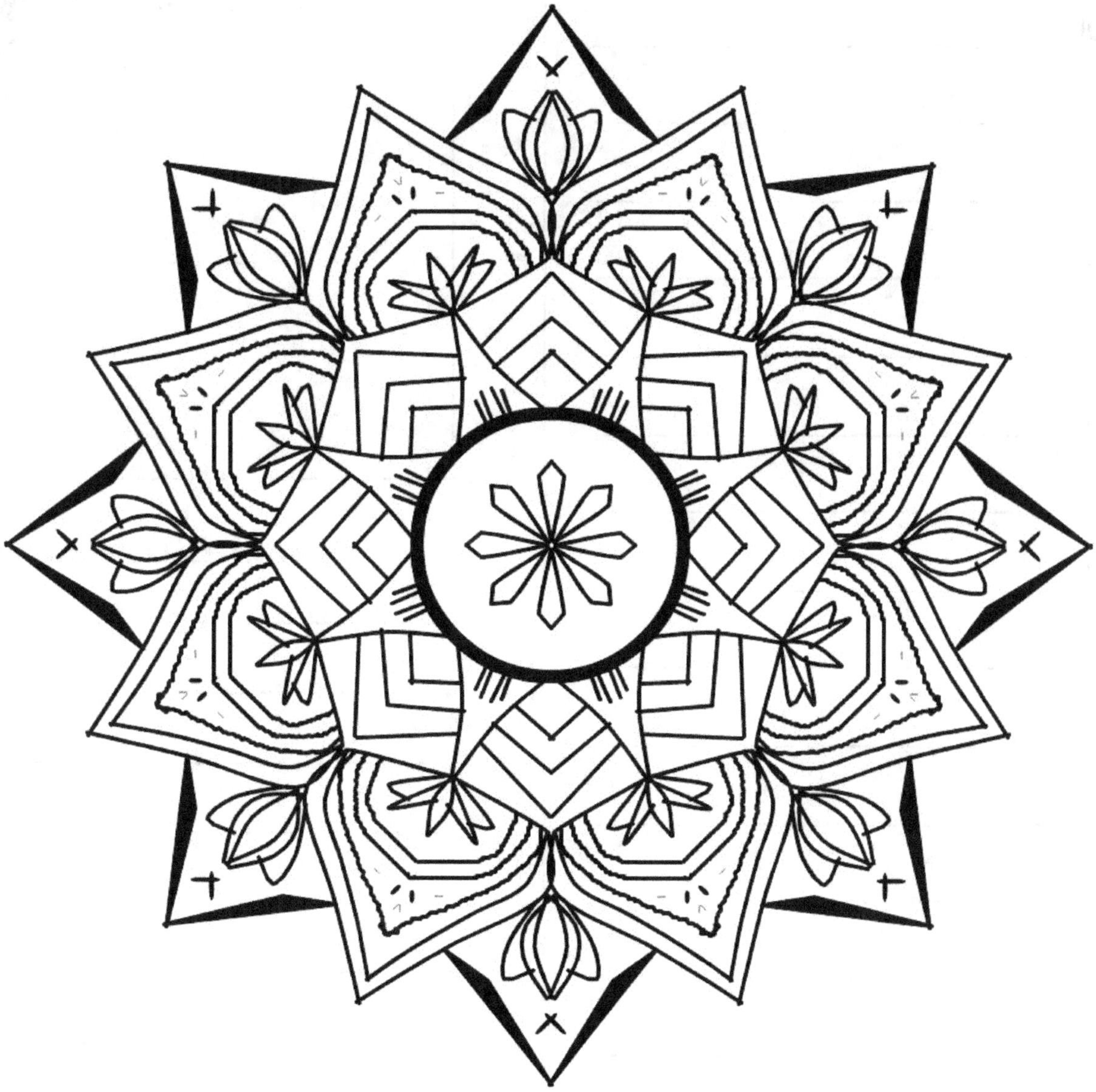

Day Seventeen _______

Time	
5:00	_______________
6:00	_______________
7:00	_______________
8:00	_______________
9:00	_______________
10:00	_______________
11:00	_______________
Noon	_______________
1:00	_______________
2:00	_______________
3:00	_______________
4:00	_______________
5:00	_______________
6:00	_______________
7:00	_______________
8:00	_______________
9:00	_______________
10:00	_______________
11:00	_______________
Midnight	_______________

top priorities for today

____
____
____
____
____

Today's victories

What makes you happy?

____
____
____
____
____
____

The Stella Society Training

Exercise	Set 1	Set 2	Set 3	Set 4	Set 5	notes

Time started: _______________   Time ended: _______________

Location: ____

Feelings before training: 

Feelings after training

NUTRITION

Meal 1

time eaten: _________

Meal 2

time eaten: _________

Meal 3

time eaten: _________

Meal 4

time eaten: _________

Meal 5

time eaten: _________

Hydration

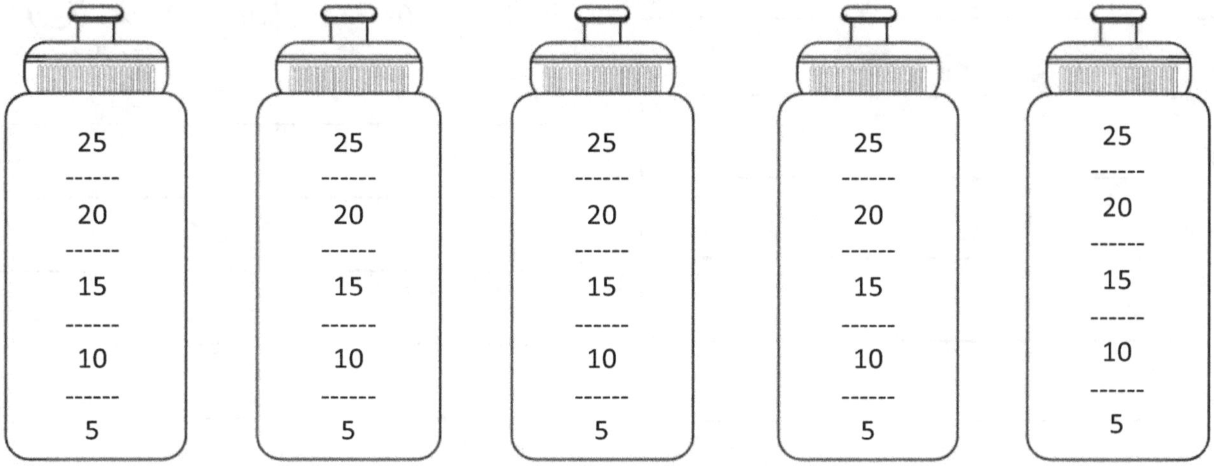

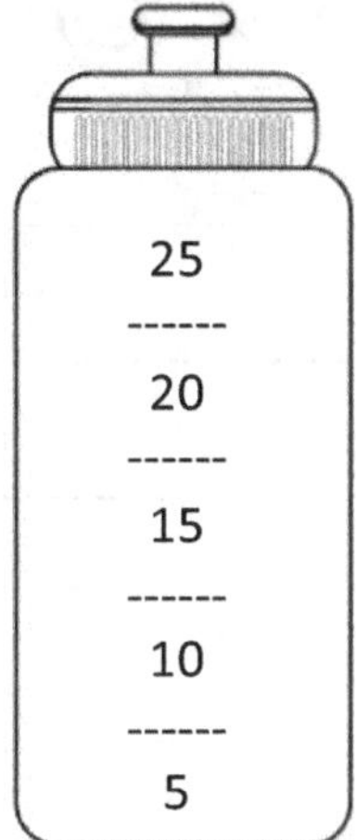
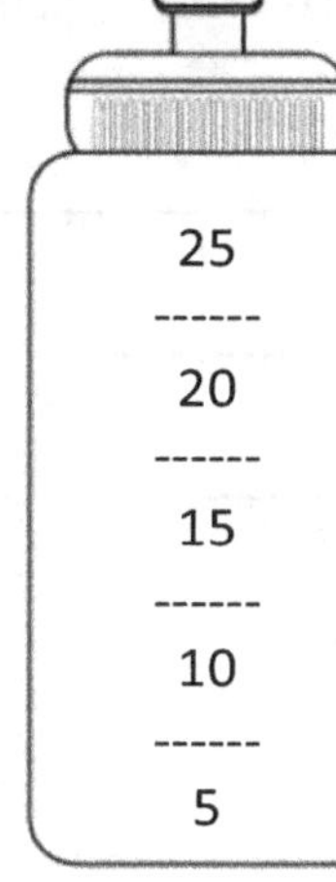
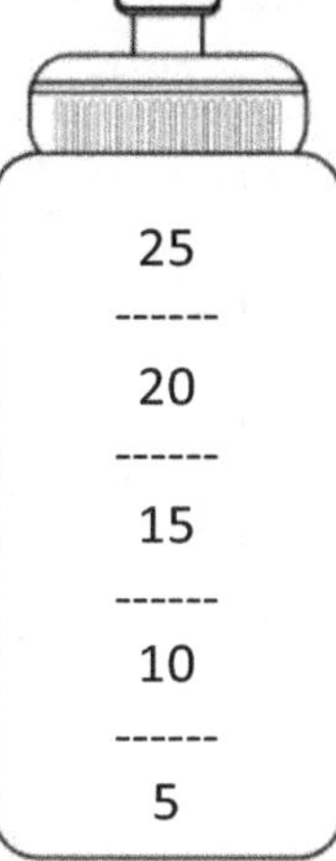

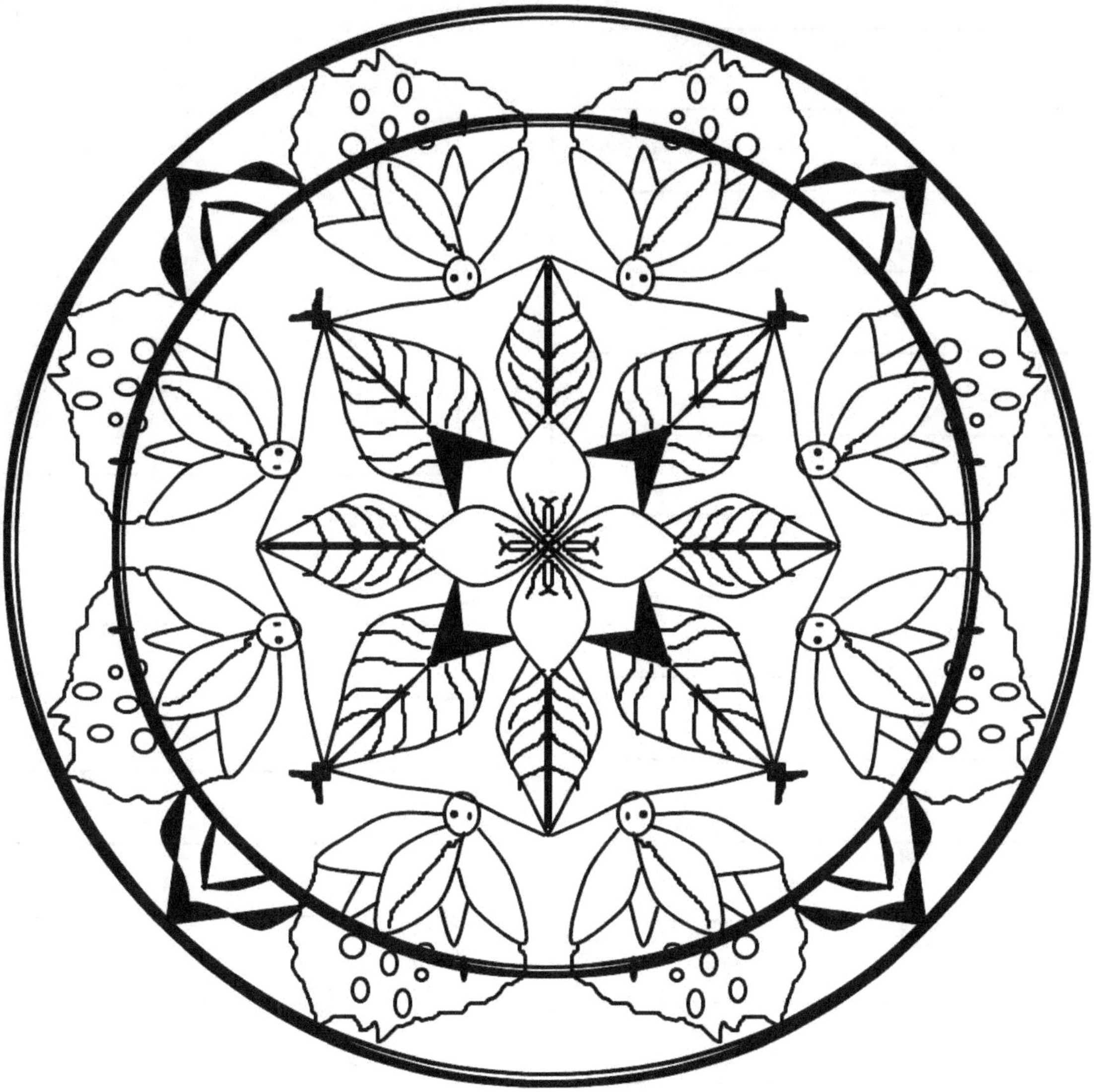

Day Eighteen _______

5:00 _________________________

6:00 _________________________

7:00 _________________________

8:00 _________________________

9:00 _________________________

10:00 ________________________

11:00 ________________________

Noon _________________________

1:00 _________________________

2:00 _________________________

3:00 _________________________

4:00 _________________________

5:00 _________________________

6:00 _________________________

7:00 _________________________

8:00 _________________________

9:00 _________________________

10:00 ________________________

11:00 ________________________

Midnight _____________________

Today's victories

Where will you shine your
light this week?

The Stella Society Training

Exercise	Set 1	Set 2	Set 3	Set 4	Set 5	notes

Time started: _____________ Time ended: _______________

Location: ____

Feelings before training:      

Feelings after training

NUTRITION

Meal 1

time eaten: _________

Meal 2

time eaten: _________

Meal 3

time eaten: _________

Meal 4

time eaten: _________

Meal 5

time eaten: _________

Hydration

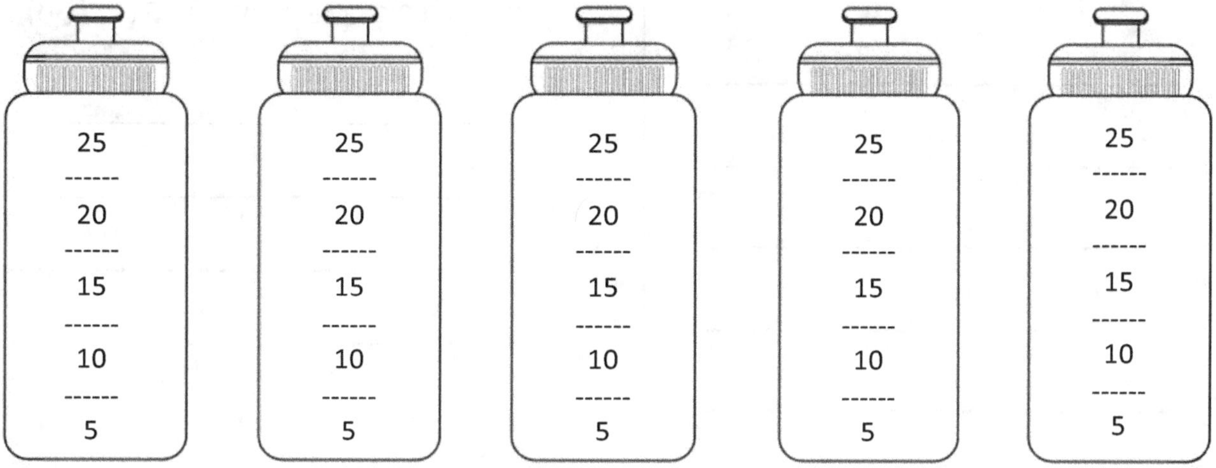

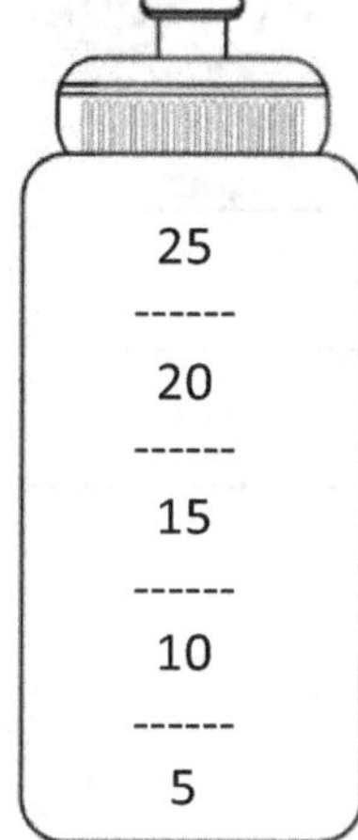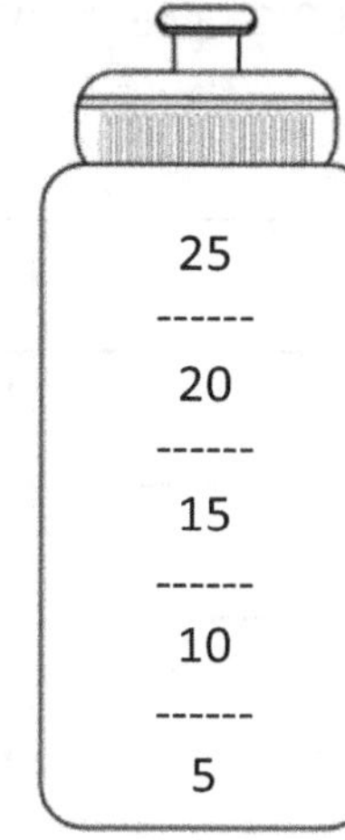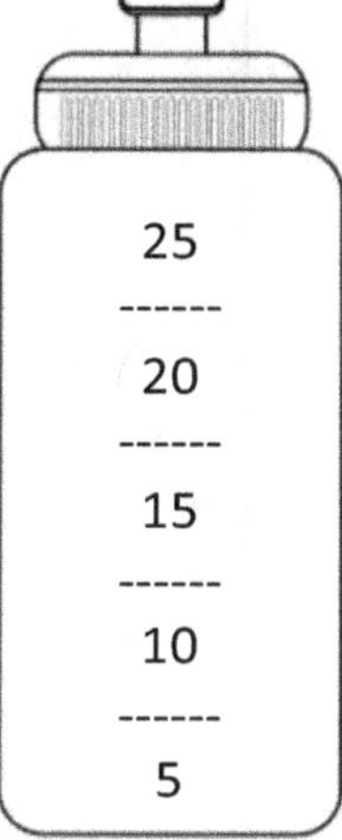

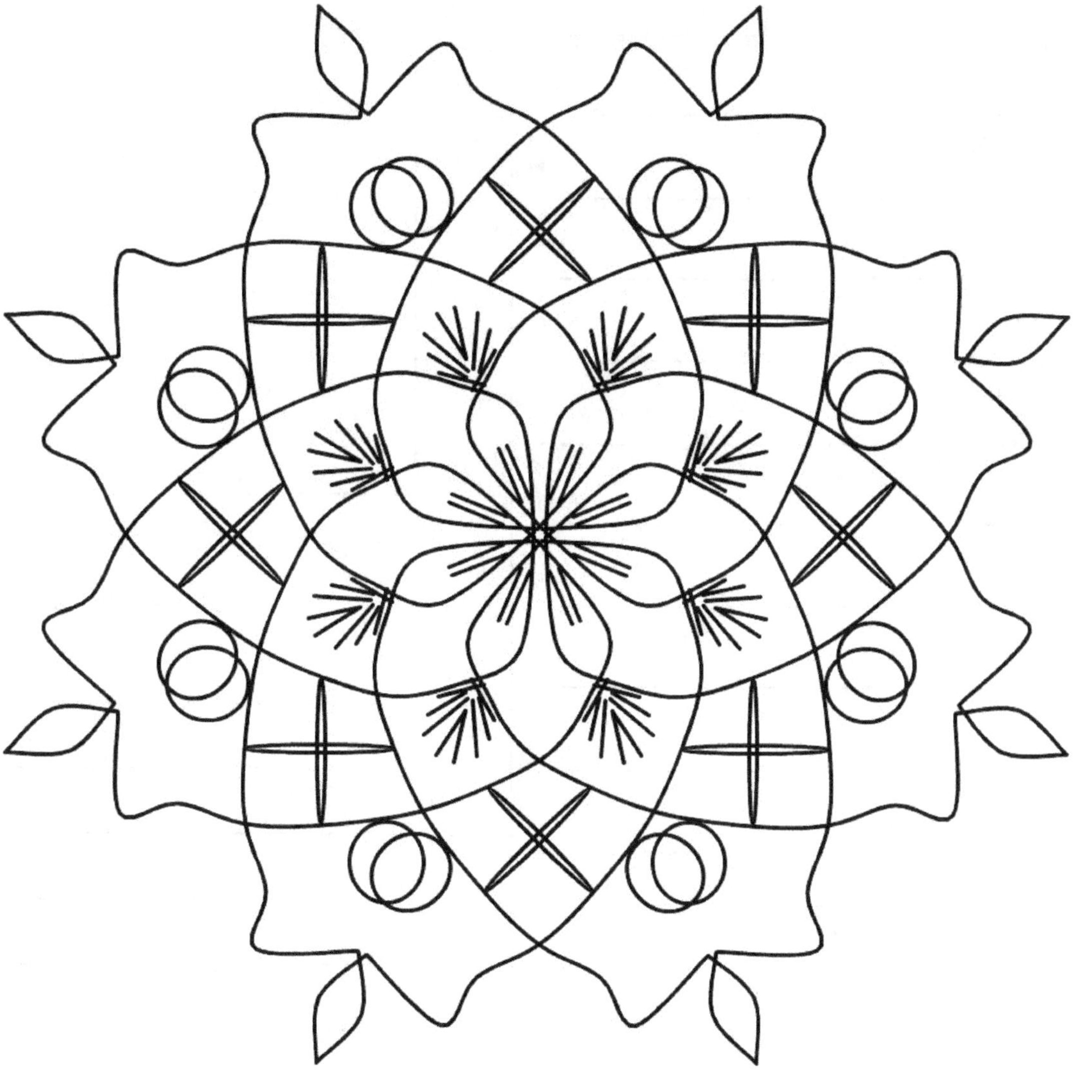

Day Nineteen ______

5:00 ______________________

6:00 ______________________

7:00 ______________________

8:00 ______________________

9:00 ______________________

10:00 ______________________

11:00 ______________________

Noon ______________________

1:00 ______________________

2:00 ______________________

3:00 ______________________

4:00 ______________________

5:00 ______________________

6:00 ______________________

7:00 ______________________

8:00 ______________________

9:00 ______________________

10:00 ______________________

11:00 ______________________

Midnight ______________________

top priorities for today

Today's victories

You are charming, how will you show it?

The Stella Society Training

Exercise	Set 1	Set 2	Set 3	Set 4	Set 5	notes

Time started: _______________   Time ended: _______________

Location: ____

Feelings before training: 🙂 😐 🙁 😝 😠 😟 😇 😎

Feelings after training 🙂 😐 🙁 😝 😠 😟 😇 😎

NUTRITION

Meal 1
time eaten: _________

Meal 2
time eaten: _________

Meal 3
time eaten: _________

Meal 4
time eaten: _________

Meal 5
time eaten: _________

Hydration

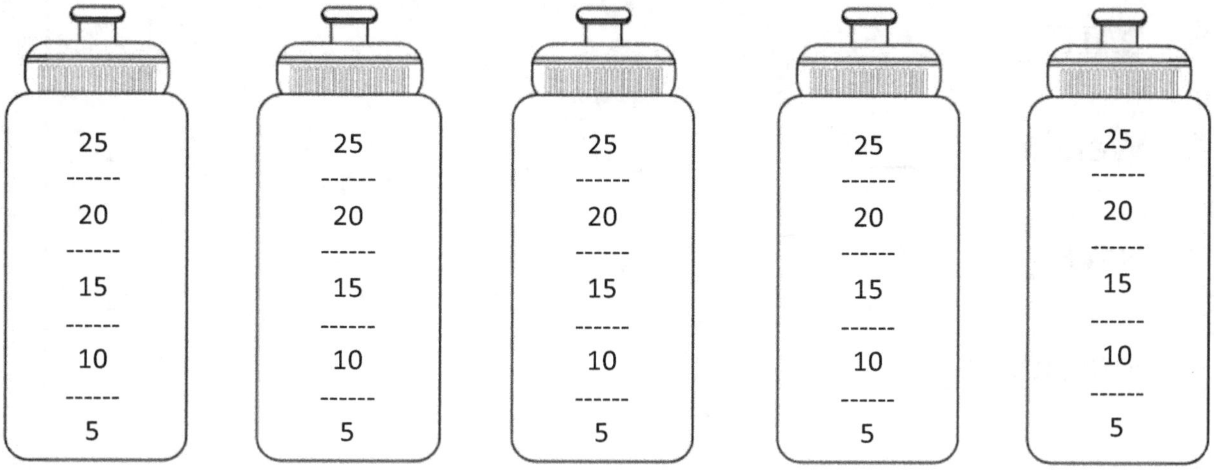

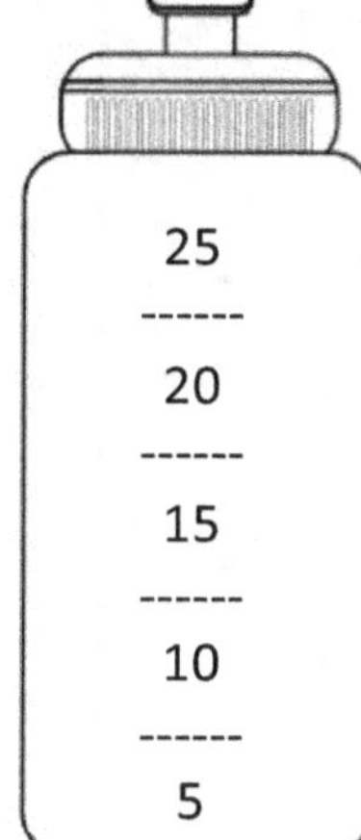
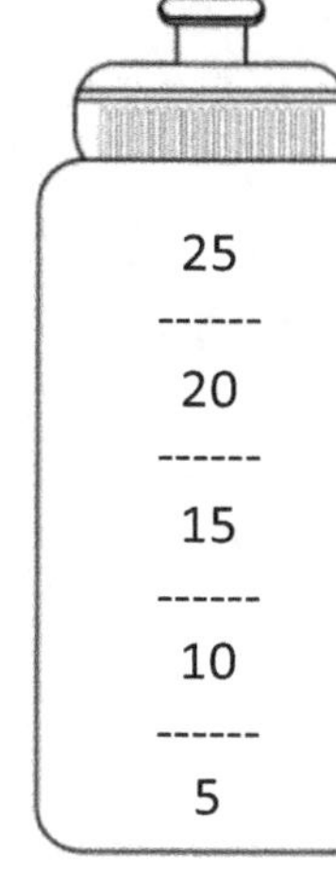

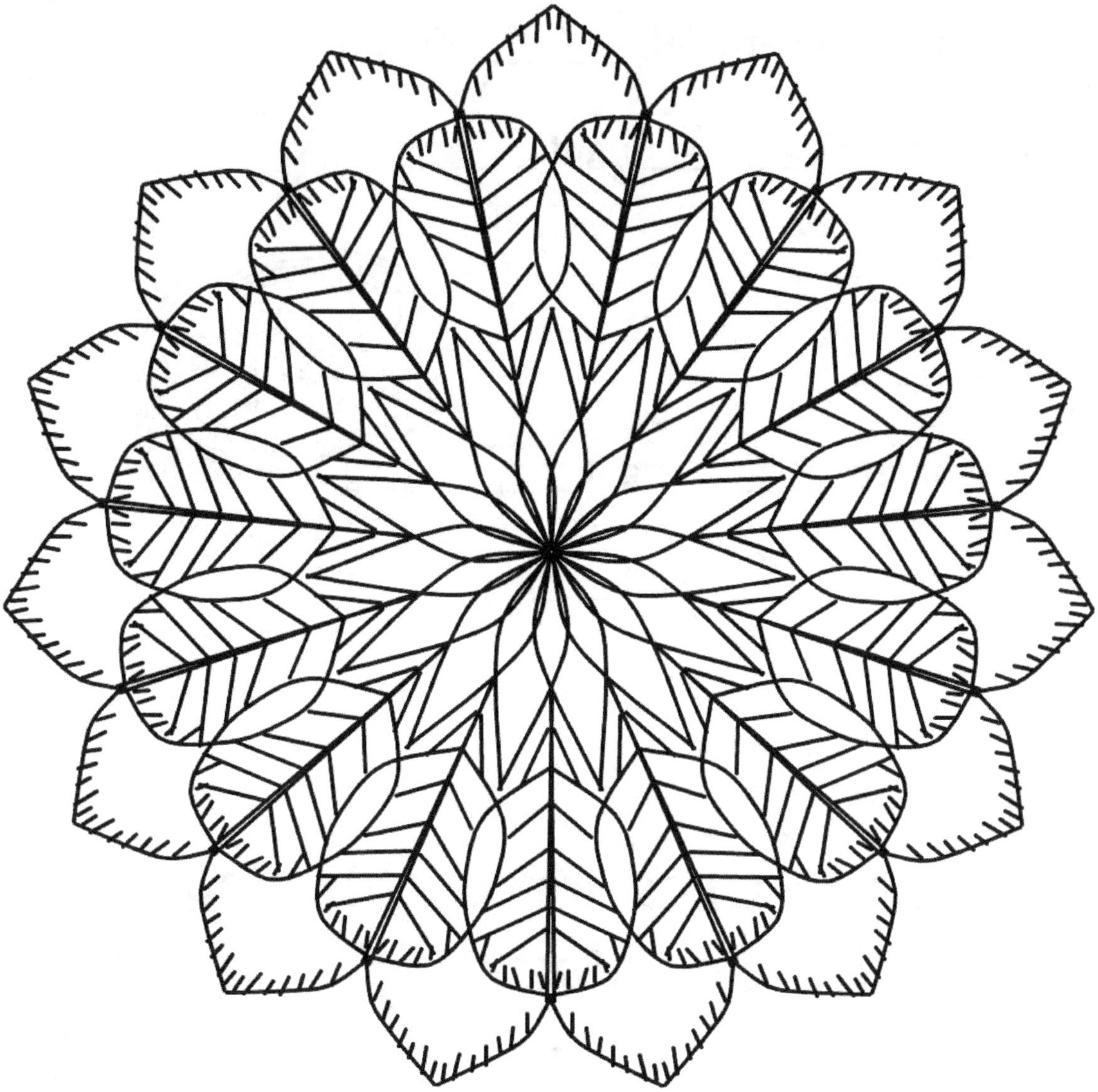

Measurements

DATE: ___________

Weight: _______

Neck _______

Shoulders _______

Chest _______

Bicep / upper arm left _________ right _______

Forearm left _______ right _______

Waist _______

Hips _______

Thighs left _______ right _____

Calf left _______ right _______

P R O G R E S S

C H E C K

Food, Like Your Money,
Should Be Working For You

Day Twenty _______

5:00 _______________________

6:00 _______________________

7:00 _______________________

8:00 _______________________

9:00 _______________________

10:00 _______________________

11:00 _______________________

Noon _______________________

1:00 _______________________

2:00 _______________________

3:00 _______________________

4:00 _______________________

5:00 _______________________

6:00 _______________________

7:00 _______________________

8:00 _______________________

9:00 _______________________

10:00 _______________________

11:00 _______________________

Midnight _______________________

top priorities for today

____
____
____
____
____

Today's victories

What is your level of understanding
difficult situations?

____
____
____
____
____
____

The Stella Society Workout

Exercise	Set 1	Set 2	Set 3	Set 4	Set 5	notes

Time started: _____________ Time ended: ______________

Location: ____

Feelings before training:

Feelings after training

NUTRITION

Meal 1

time eaten: _________

Meal 2

time eaten: _________

Meal 3

time eaten: _________

Meal 4

time eaten: _________

Meal 5

time eaten: _________

Hydration

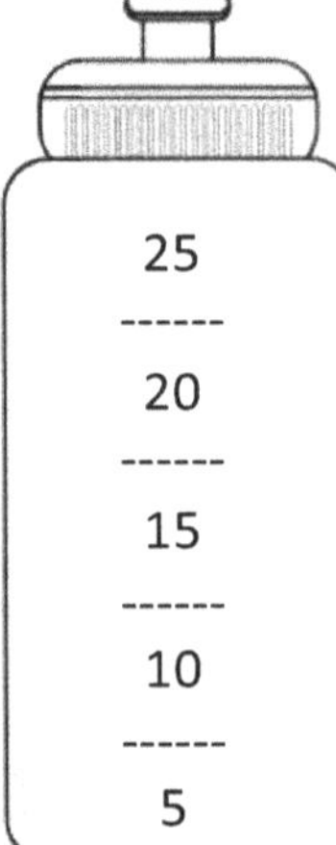

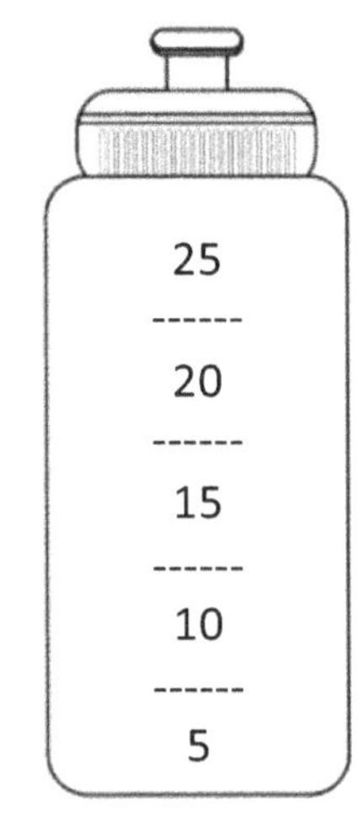

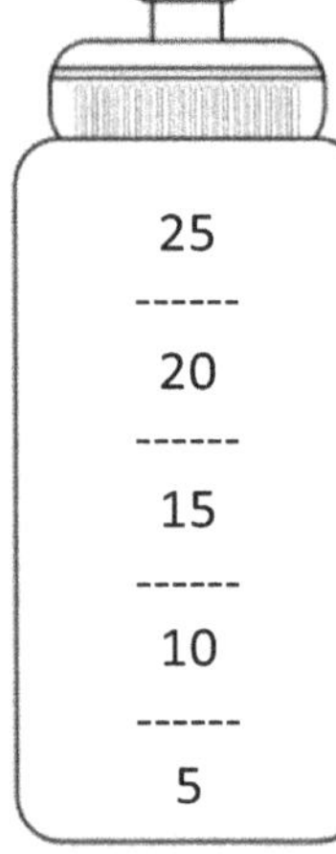

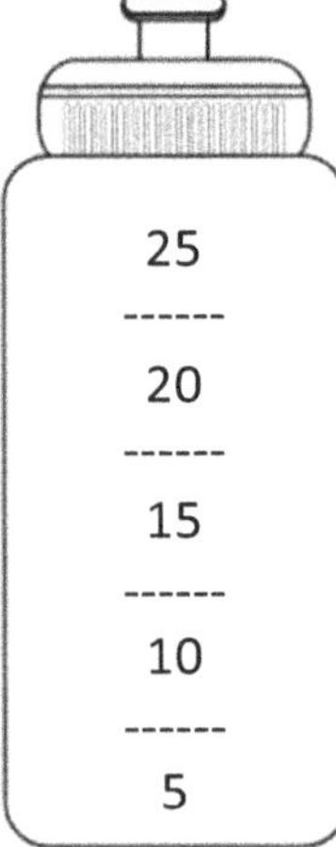

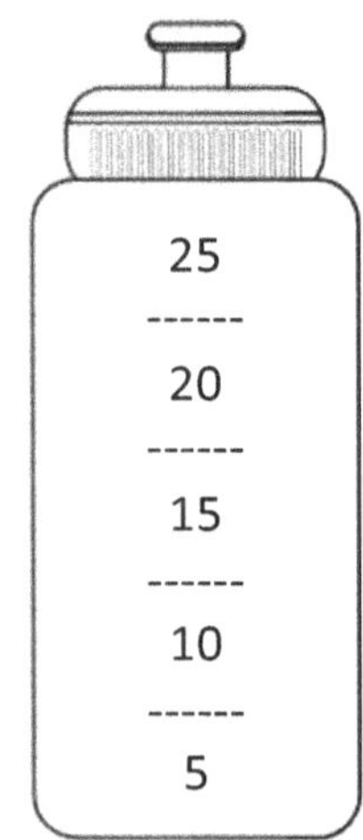

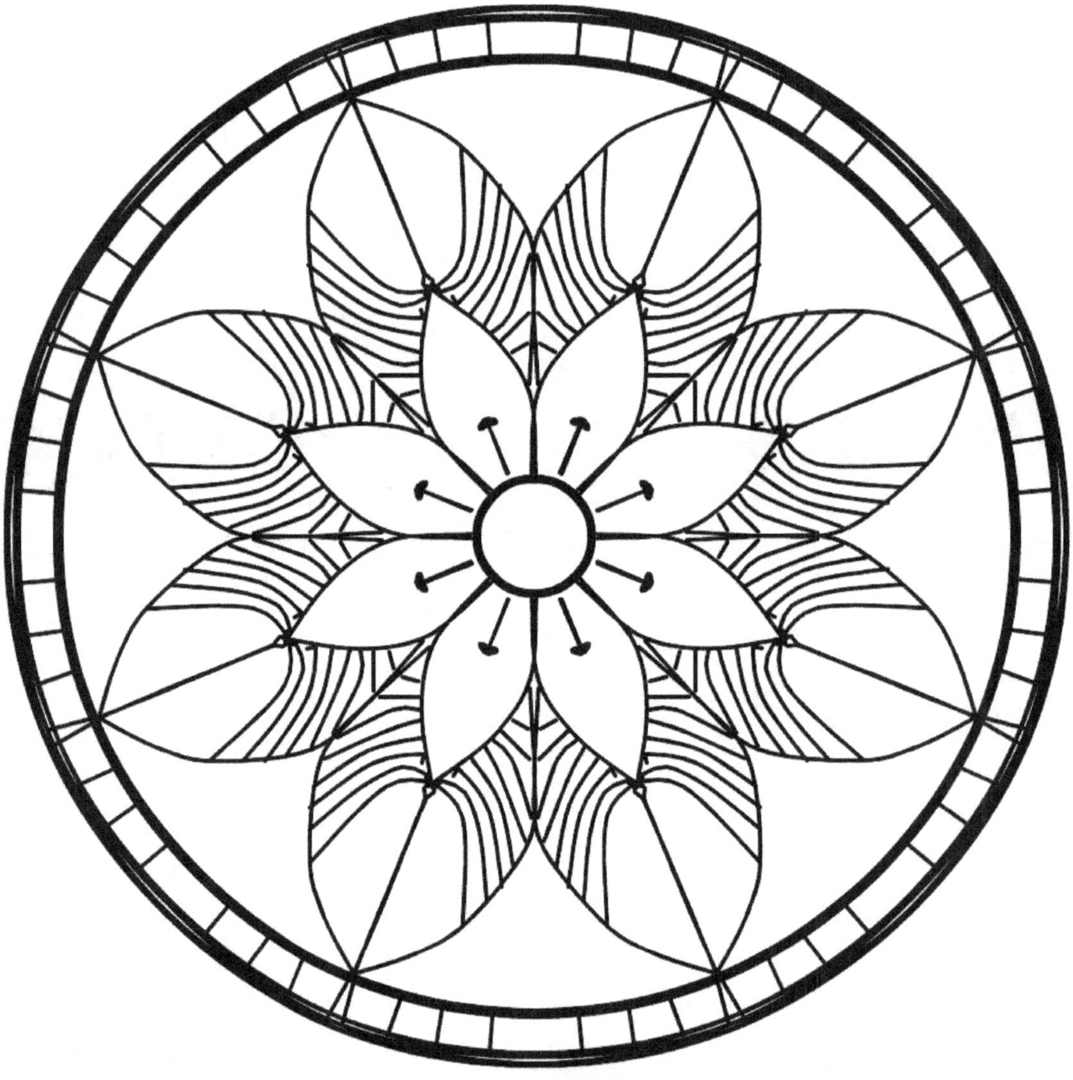

Day Twenty-one ______

5:00	__________________
6:00	__________________
7:00	__________________
8:00	__________________
9:00	__________________
10:00	__________________
11:00	__________________
Noon	__________________
1:00	__________________
2:00	__________________
3:00	__________________
4:00	__________________
5:00	__________________
6:00	__________________
7:00	__________________
8:00	__________________
9:00	__________________
10:00	__________________
11:00	__________________
Midnight	__________________

top priorities for today 🎯

____

____

____

____

____

Today's victories 🏆

How much can you endure?

____

____

____

____

____

____

____

The *Stella Society* Workout

Exercise	Set 1	Set 2	Set 3	Set 4	Set 5	notes

Time started: _____________ Time ended: _____________

Location: _______________________________________

Feelings before training:

Feelings after training

NUTRITION

Meal 1

time eaten: _________

Meal 2

time eaten: _________

Meal 3

time eaten: _________

Meal 4

time eaten: _________

Meal 5

time eaten: _________

Hydration

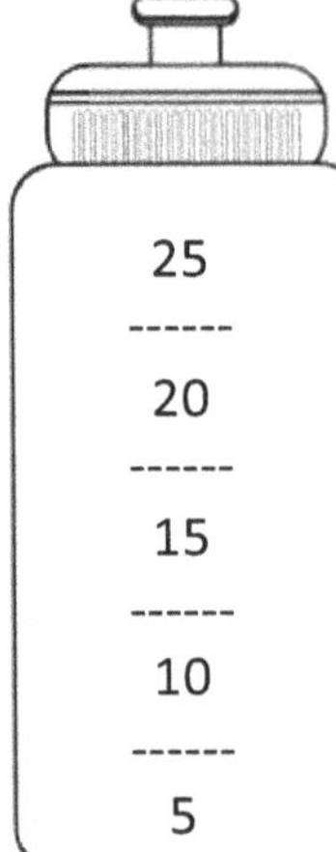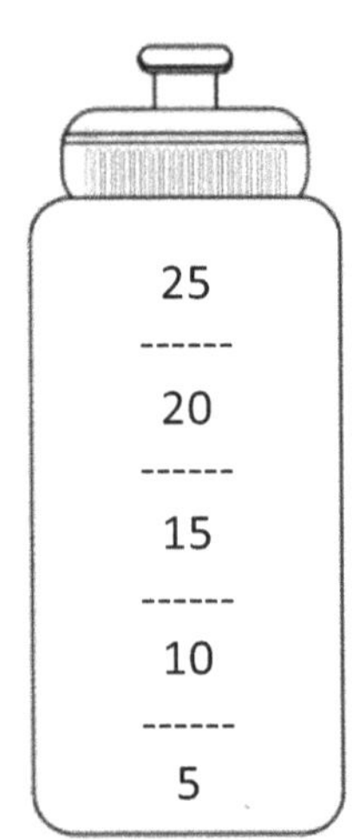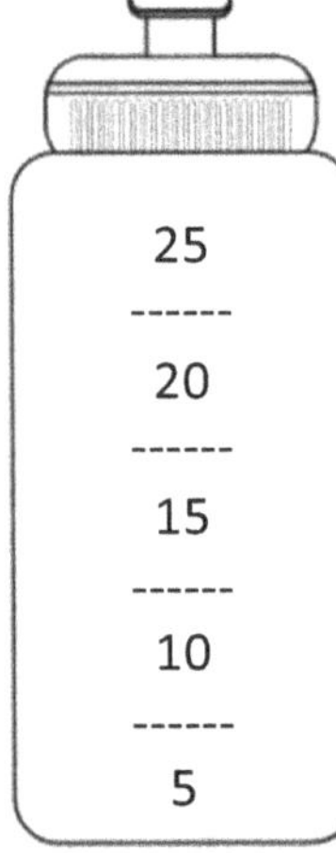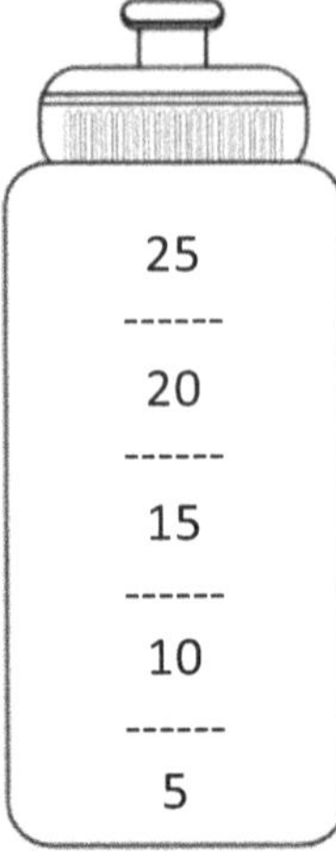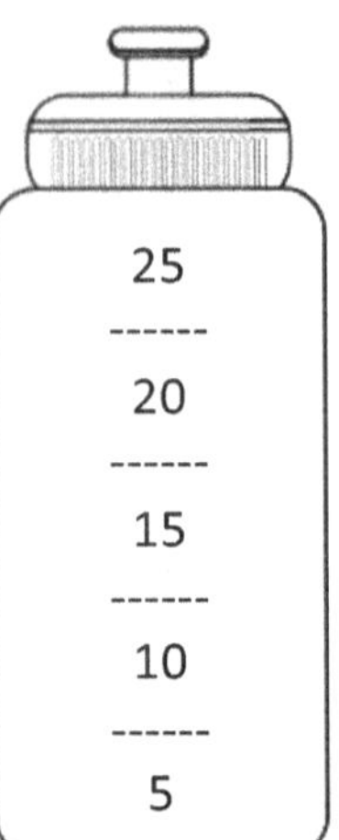

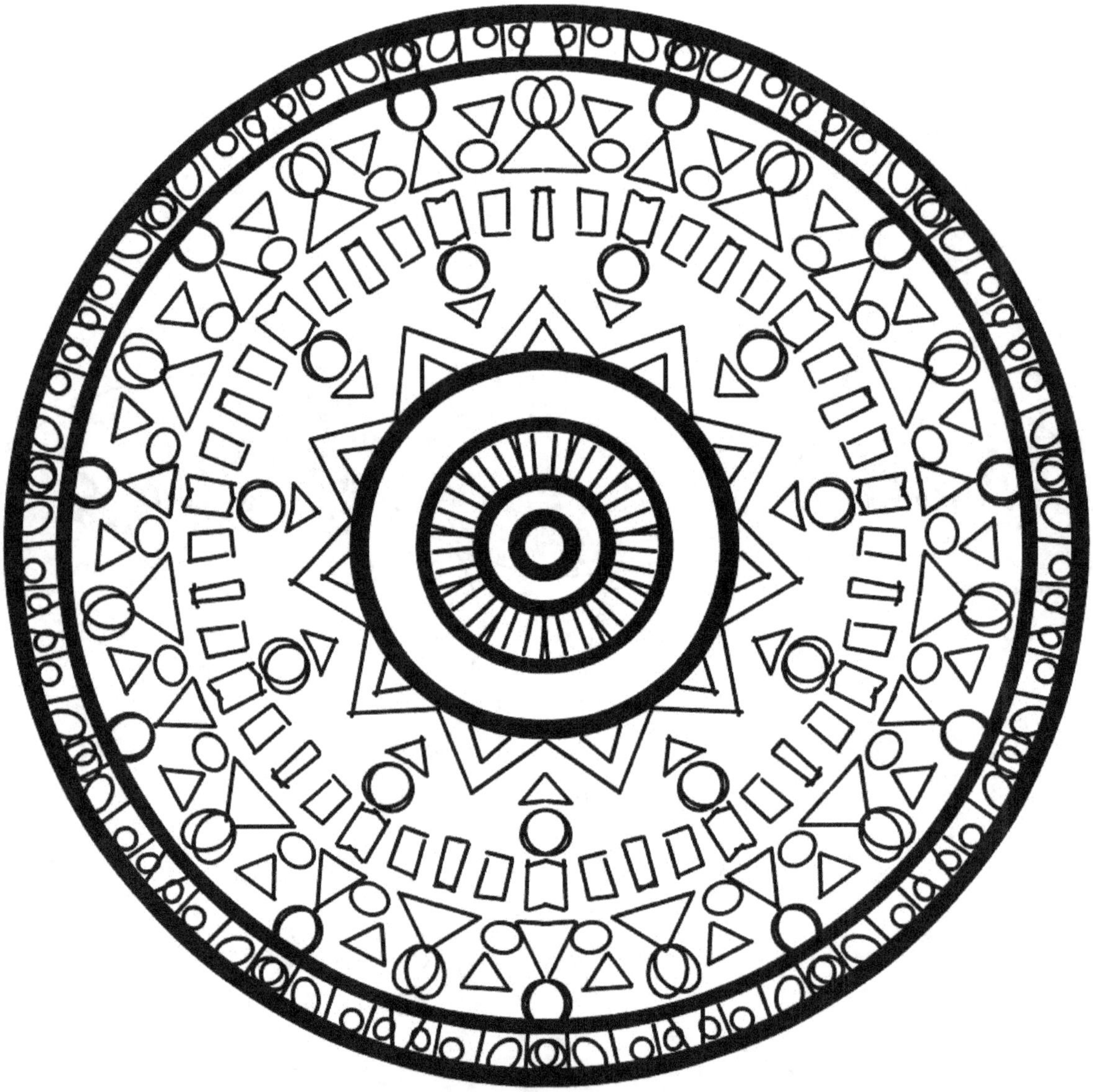

Day Twenty-two _______

5:00	_______________________
6:00	_______________________
7:00	_______________________
8:00	_______________________
9:00	_______________________
10:00	_______________________
11:00	_______________________
Noon	_______________________
1:00	_______________________
2:00	_______________________
3:00	_______________________
4:00	_______________________
5:00	_______________________
6:00	_______________________
7:00	_______________________
8:00	_______________________
9:00	_______________________
10:00	_______________________
11:00	_______________________
Midnight	_______________________

top priorities for today

____
____
____
____
____

Today's victories

List 5 ways to be thoughtful.

____
____
____
____
____

The *Stella Society* Workout

Exercise	Set 1	Set 2	Set 3	Set 4	Set 5	notes

Time started: _____________ Time ended: ______________

Location: ____

Feelings before training:

Feelings after training

NUTRITION

Meal 1

time eaten: _________

Meal 2

time eaten: _________

Meal 3

time eaten: _________

Meal 4

time eaten: _________

Meal 5

time eaten: _________

Hydration

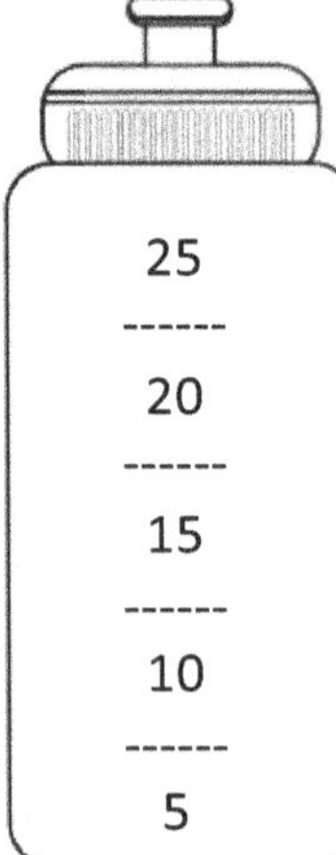

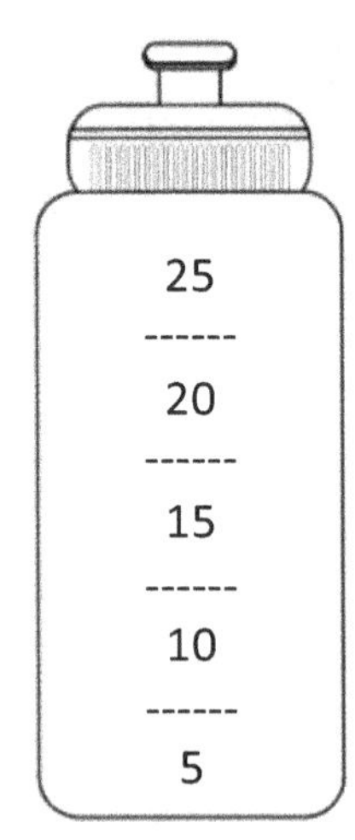

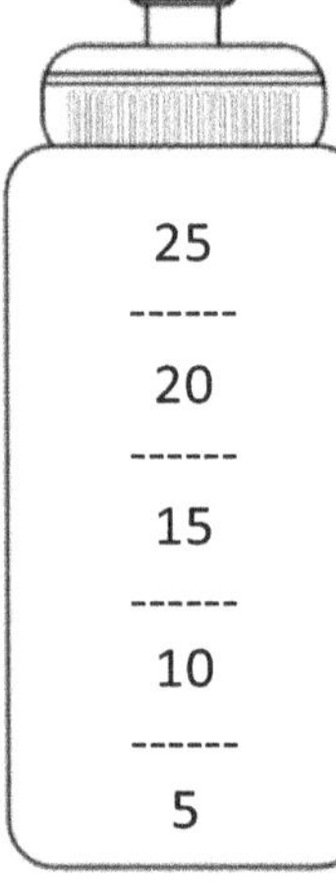

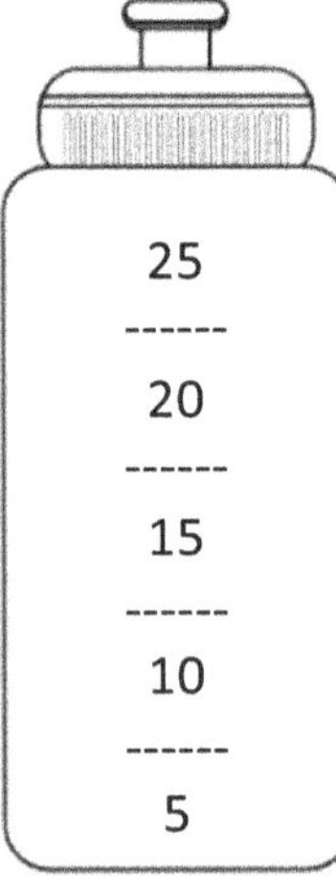

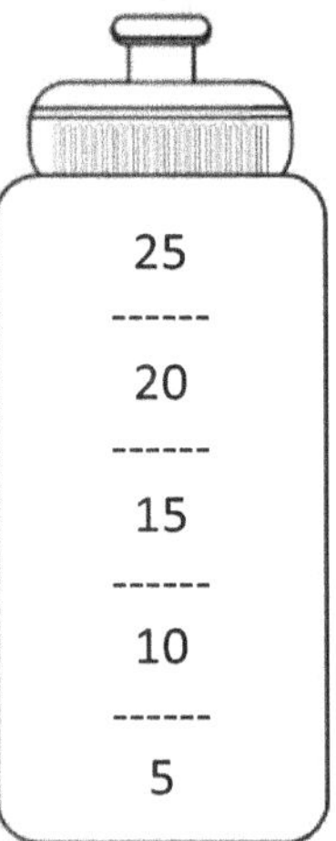

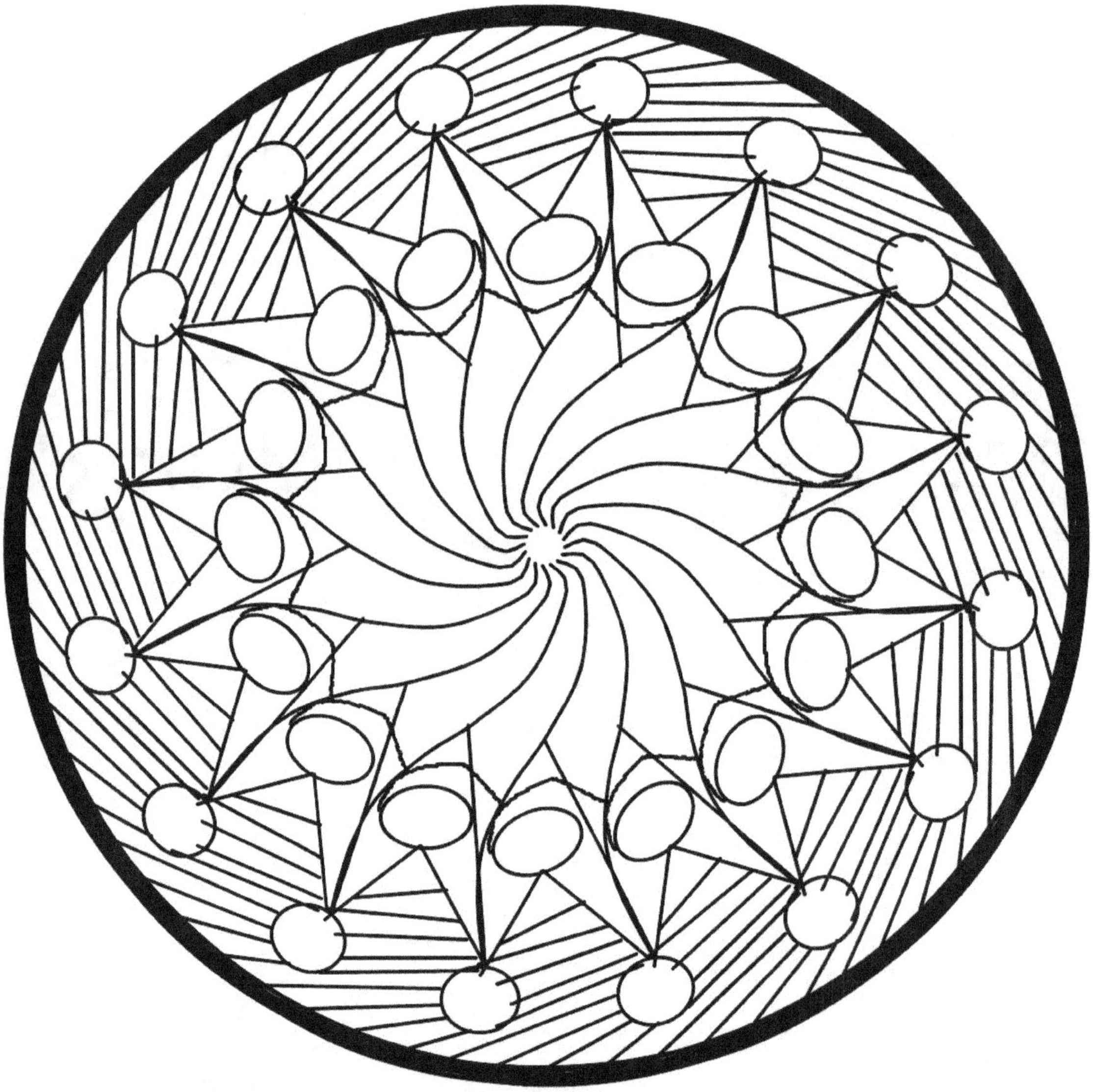

Day Twenty-three _______

5:00 _______________________

6:00 _______________________

7:00 _______________________

8:00 _______________________

9:00 _______________________

10:00 ______________________

11:00 ______________________

Noon _______________________

1:00 _______________________

2:00 _______________________

3:00 _______________________

4:00 _______________________

5:00 _______________________

6:00 _______________________

7:00 _______________________

8:00 _______________________

9:00 _______________________

10:00 ______________________

11:00 ______________________

Midnight ___________________

top priorities for today

____

____

____

____

Today's victories

Why should you be unapologetic?

____

____

____

____

____

The Stella Society Workout

Exercise	Set 1	Set 2	Set 3	Set 4	Set 5	notes

Time started: _____________   Time ended: _____________

Location: ____

Feelings before training: 🙂 😐 🙁 😝 😠 😕 😇 😎

Feelings after training 🙂 😐 🙁 😝 😠 😕 😇 😎

NUTRITION

Meal 1
time eaten: _________

Meal 2
time eaten: _________

Meal 3
time eaten: _________

Meal 4
time eaten: _________

Meal 5
time eaten: _________

Hydration

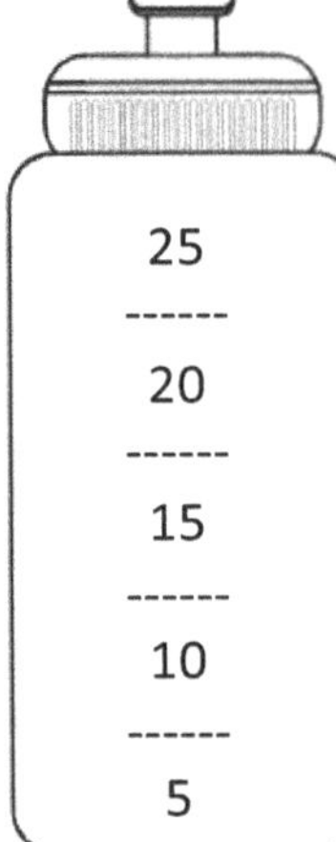

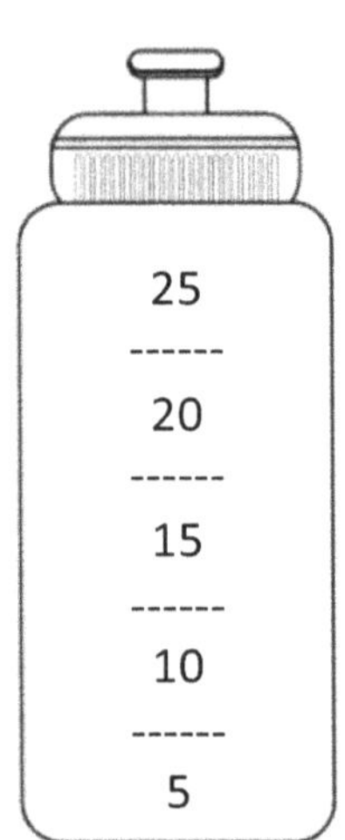

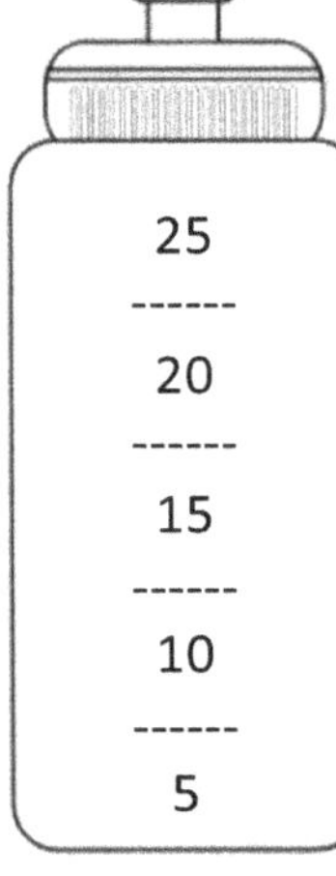

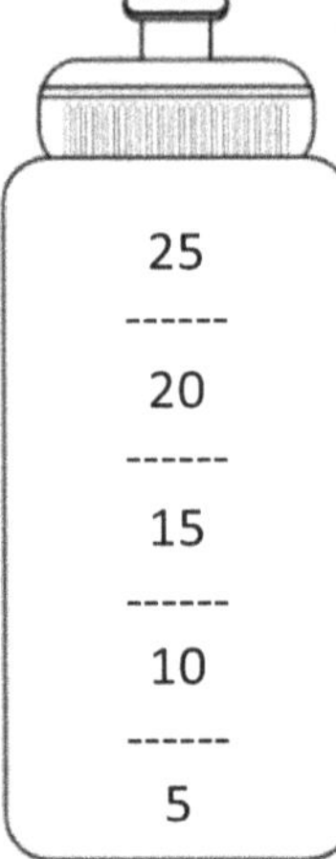

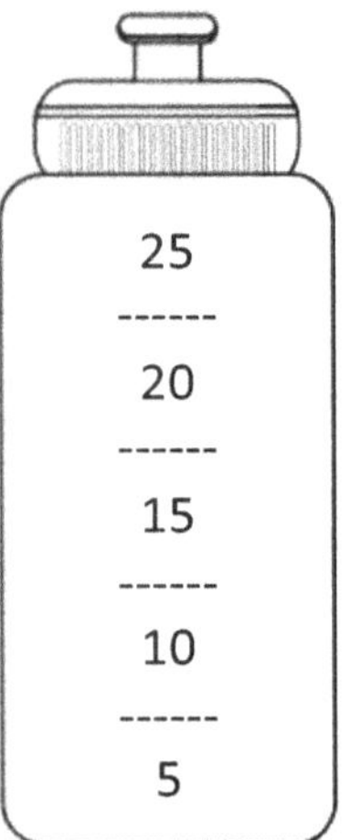

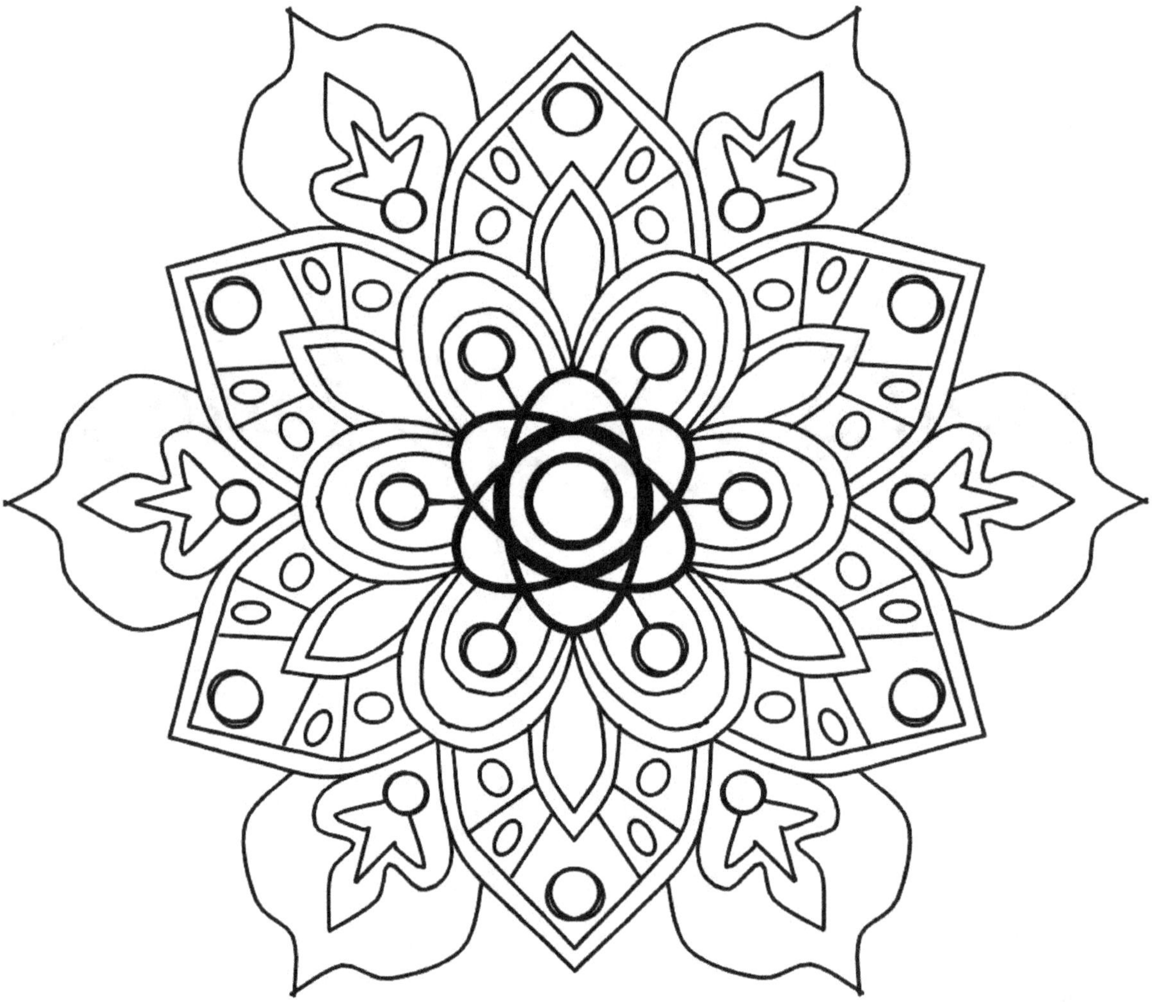

Day Twenty-four ______

5:00 __________________________

6:00 __________________________

7:00 __________________________

8:00 __________________________

9:00 __________________________

10:00 ________________________

11:00 ________________________

Noon _________________________

1:00 __________________________

2:00 __________________________

3:00 __________________________

4:00 __________________________

5:00 __________________________

6:00 __________________________

7:00 __________________________

8:00 __________________________

9:00 __________________________

10:00 ________________________

11:00 ________________________

Midnight ____________________

top priorities for today

____

____

____

____

Today's victories

What can you set on fire
with your fierceness?

____

____

____

____

____

The Stella Society Workout

Exercise	Set 1	Set 2	Set 3	Set 4	Set 5	notes

Time started: _______________   Time ended: _______________

Location: ____

Feelings before training:

Feelings after training

NUTRITION

Meal 1
time eaten: _________

Meal 2
time eaten: _________

Meal 3
time eaten: _________

Meal 4
time eaten: _________

Meal 5
time eaten: _________

Hydration

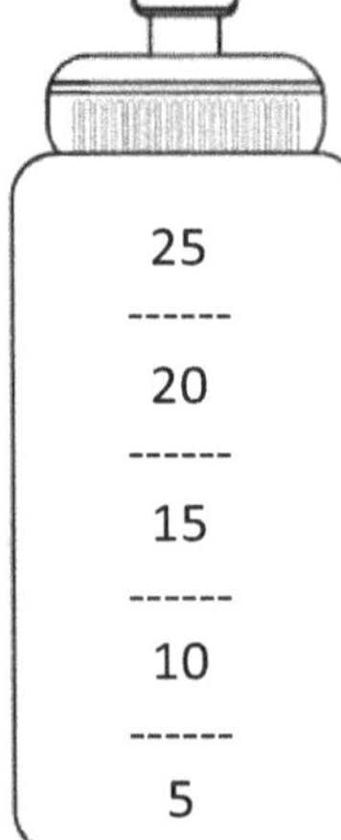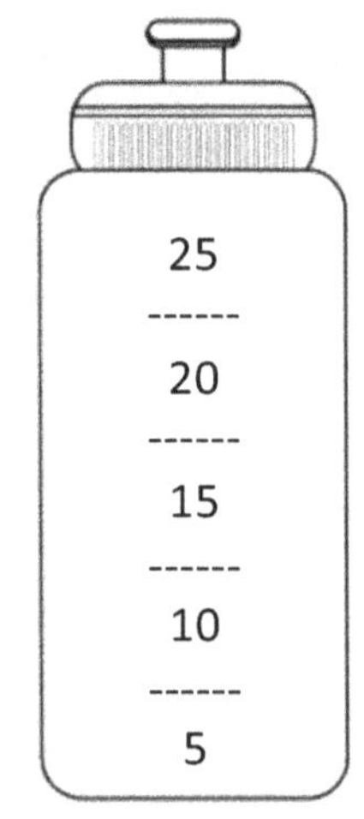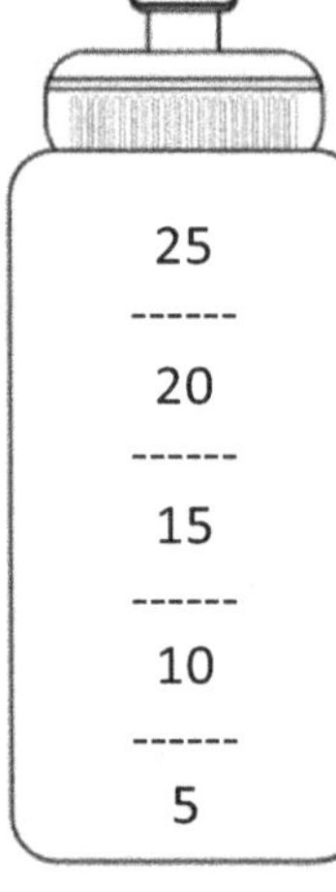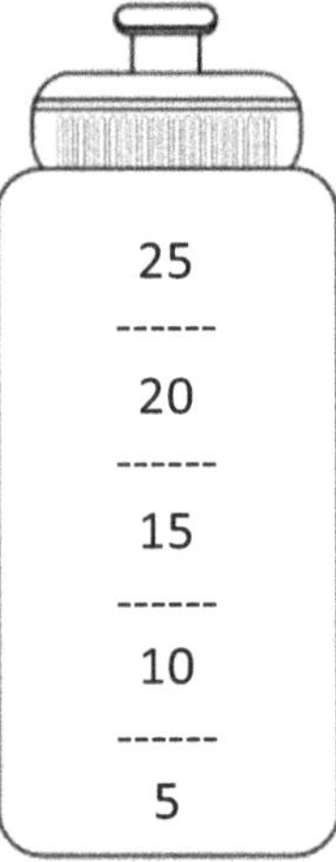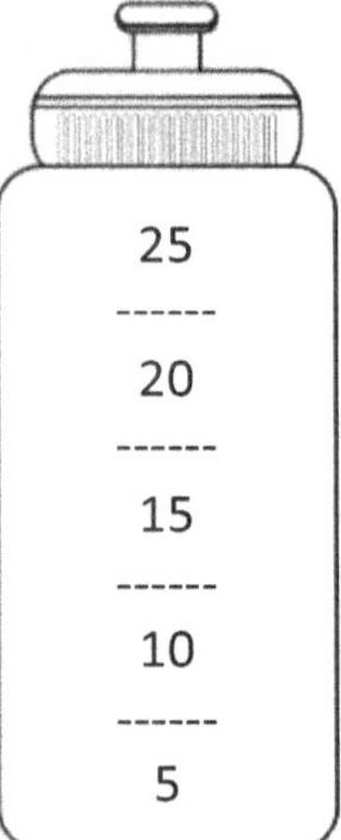

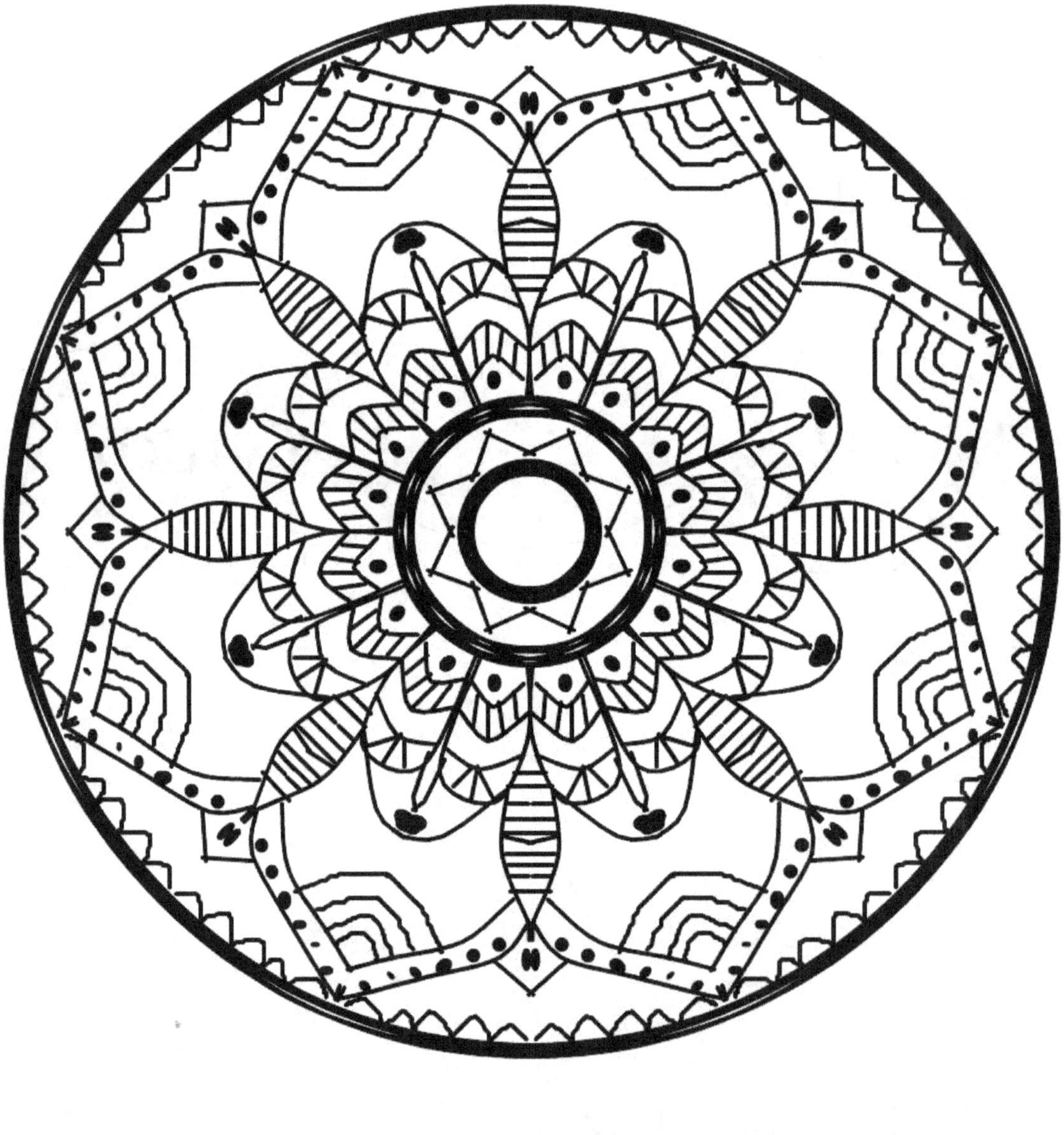

Day Twenty-five _______

5:00	_______________
6:00	_______________
7:00	_______________
8:00	_______________
9:00	_______________
10:00	_______________
11:00	_______________
Noon	_______________
1:00	_______________
2:00	_______________
3:00	_______________
4:00	_______________
5:00	_______________
6:00	_______________
7:00	_______________
8:00	_______________
9:00	_______________
10:00	_______________
11:00	_______________
Midnight	_______________

top priorities for today 🎯

____

____

____

____

Today's victories 🏆

Make it your mission to stay positive. Write your positive mission statement.

____

____

____

____

____

The Stella Society Workout

Exercise	Set 1	Set 2	Set 3	Set 4	Set 5	notes

Time started: _____________   Time ended: _____________

Location: ____

Feelings before training:

Feelings after training

NUTRITION

Meal 1
time eaten: _________

Meal 2
time eaten: _________

Meal 3
time eaten: _________

Meal 4
time eaten: _________

Meal 5
time eaten: _________

Hydration

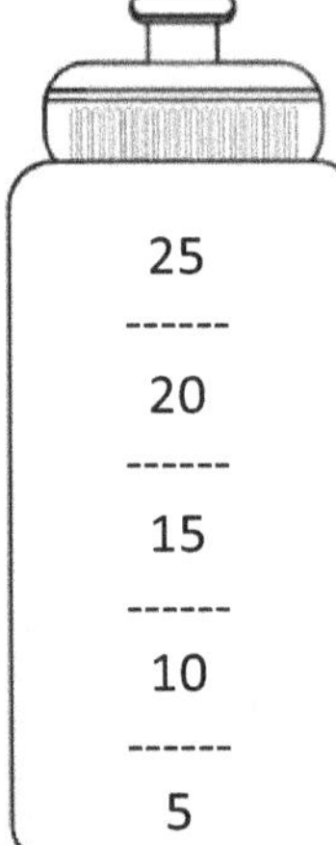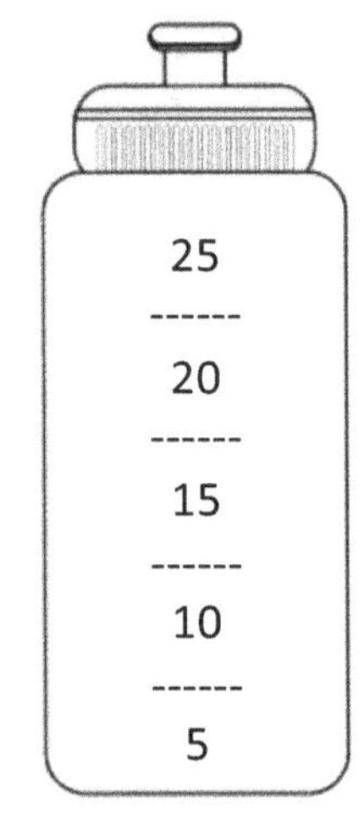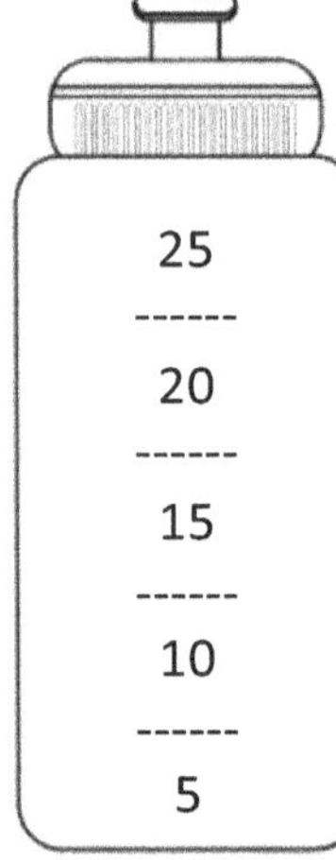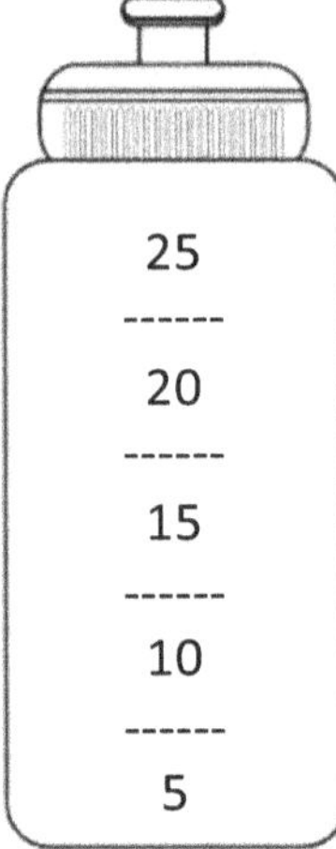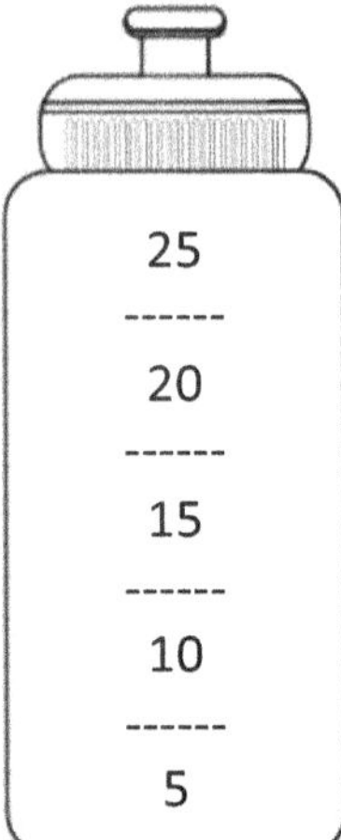

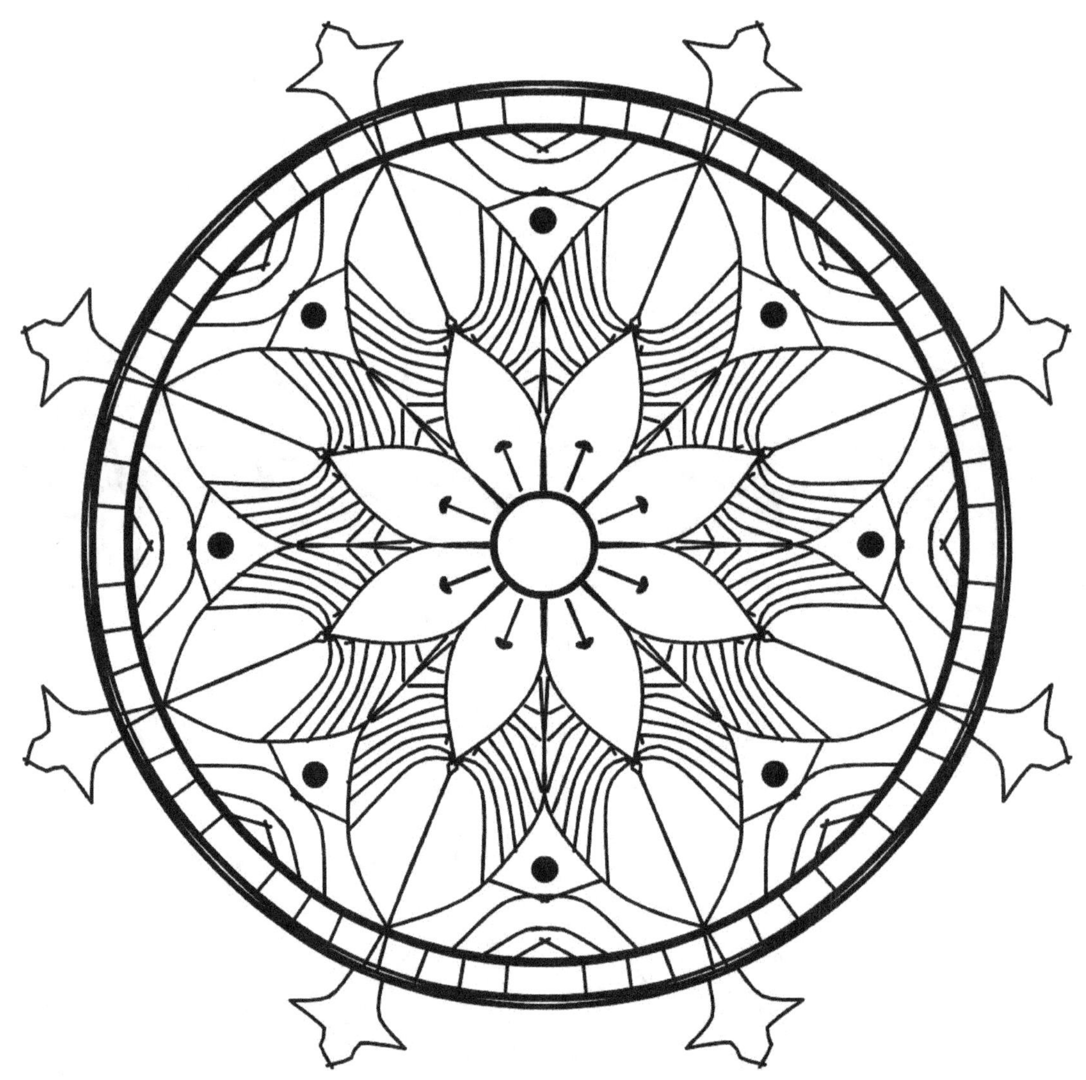

Day Twenty-six ______

5:00 ________________________

6:00 ________________________

7:00 ________________________

8:00 ________________________

9:00 ________________________

10:00 ________________________

11:00 ________________________

Noon ________________________

1:00 ________________________

2:00 ________________________

3:00 ________________________

4:00 ________________________

5:00 ________________________

6:00 ________________________

7:00 ________________________

8:00 ________________________

9:00 ________________________

10:00 ________________________

11:00 ________________________

Midnight ________________________

top priorities for today

Today's victories

What give you your inner energy?

The Stella Society Workout

Exercise	Set 1	Set 2	Set 3	Set 4	Set 5	notes

Time started: ________________ Time ended: ________________

Location: ____

Feelings before training:

Feelings after training

NUTRITION

Meal 1

time eaten: _________

Meal 2

time eaten: _________

Meal 3

time eaten: _________

Meal 4

time eaten: _________

Meal 5

time eaten: _________

Hydration

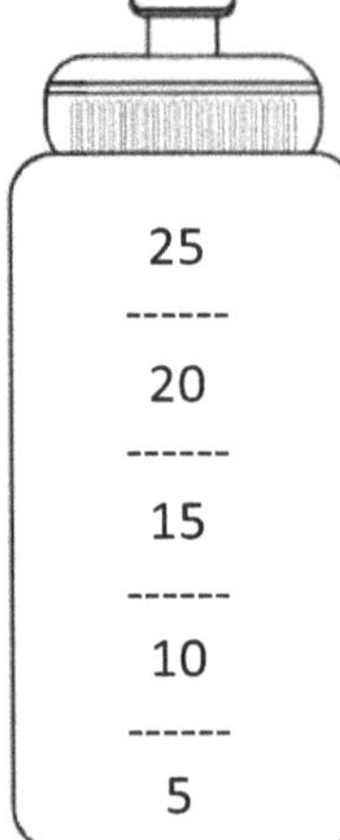

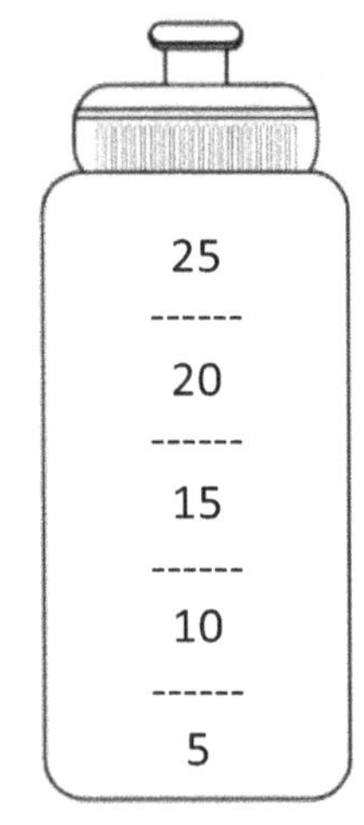

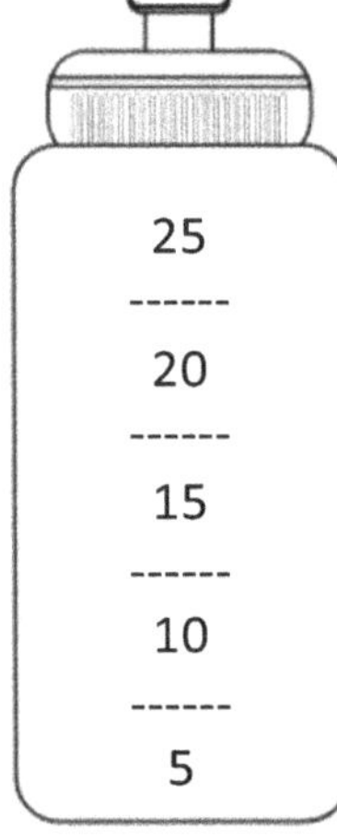

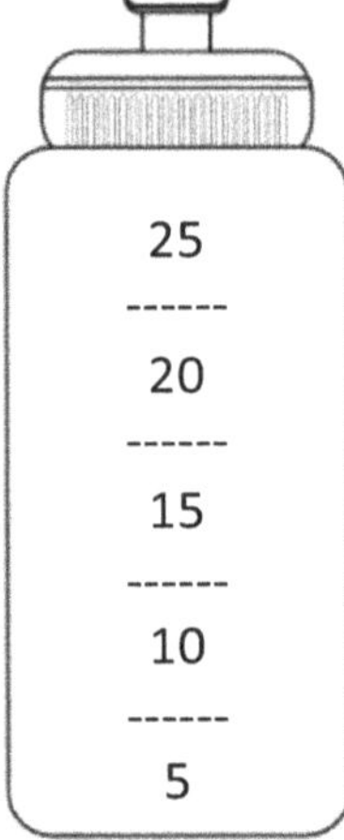

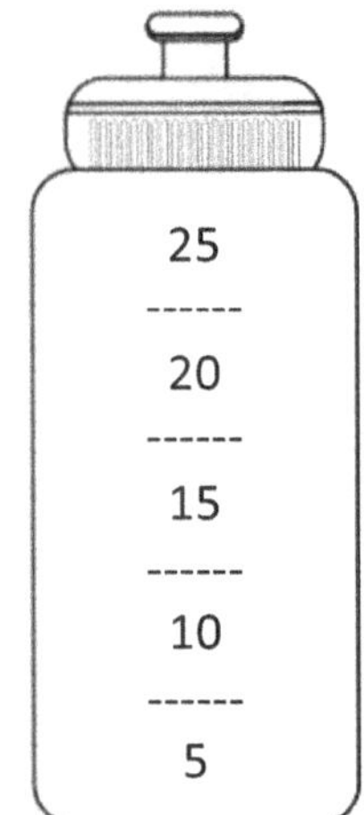

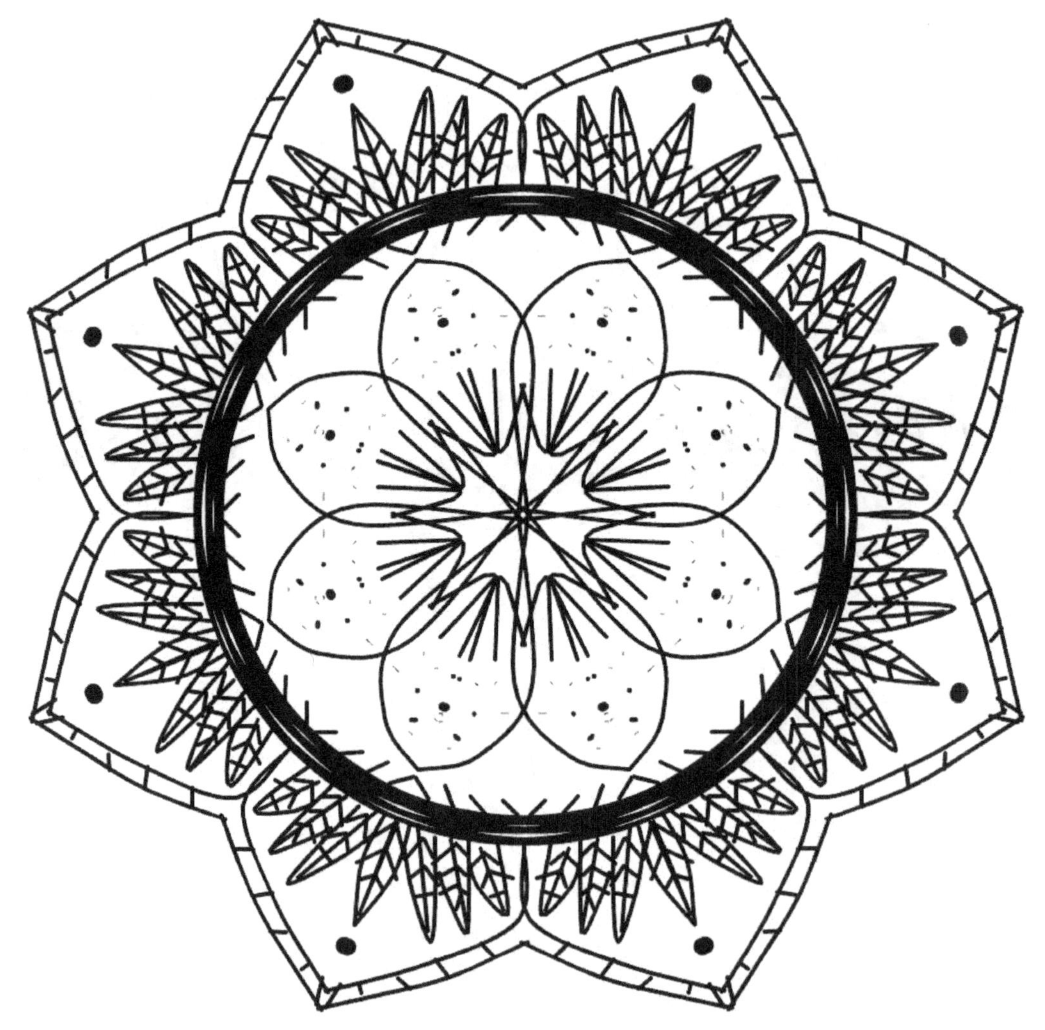

Day Twenty-seven _______

5:00 _______________________

6:00 _______________________

7:00 _______________________

8:00 _______________________

9:00 _______________________

10:00 ______________________

11:00 ______________________

Noon _______________________

1:00 _______________________

2:00 _______________________

3:00 _______________________

4:00 _______________________

5:00 _______________________

6:00 _______________________

7:00 _______________________

8:00 _______________________

9:00 _______________________

10:00 ______________________

11:00 ______________________

Midnight ____________________

Today's victories

What have you stopped, but
won't stop again?

The Stella Society Workout

Exercise	Set 1	Set 2	Set 3	Set 4	Set 5	notes

Time started: _______________   Time ended: _______________

Location: ____

Feelings before training:

Feelings after training

NUTRITION

Meal 1

time eaten: _________

Meal 2

time eaten: _________

Meal 3

time eaten: _________

Meal 4

time eaten: _________

Meal 5

time eaten: _________

Hydration

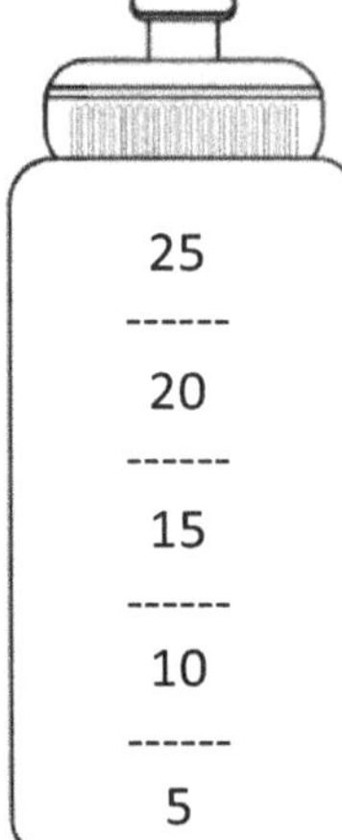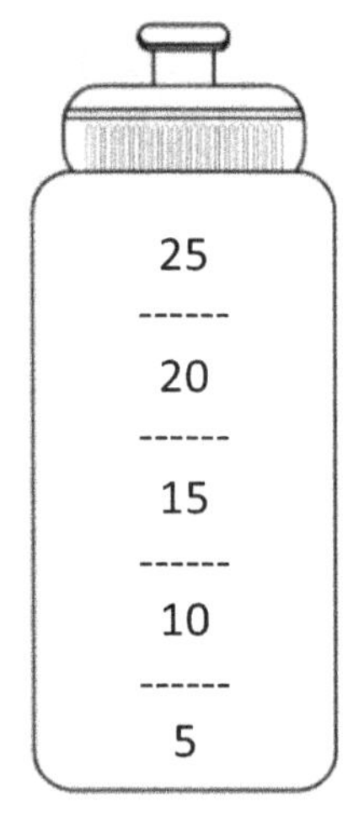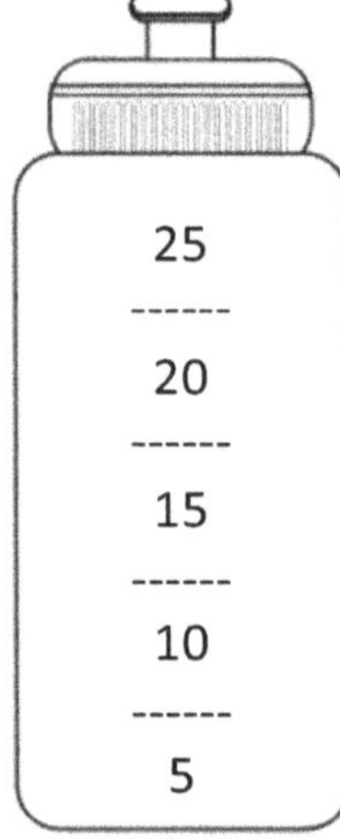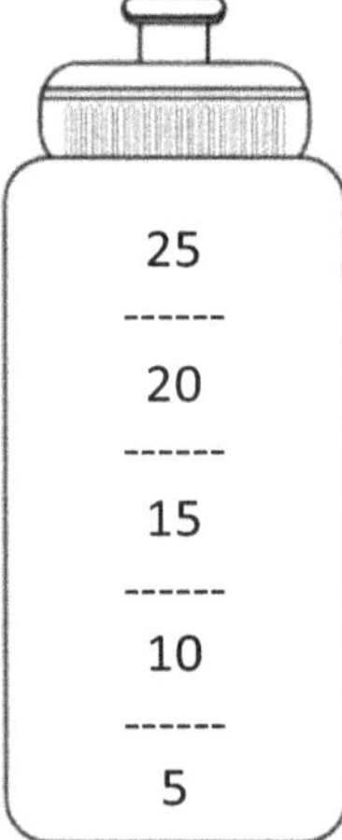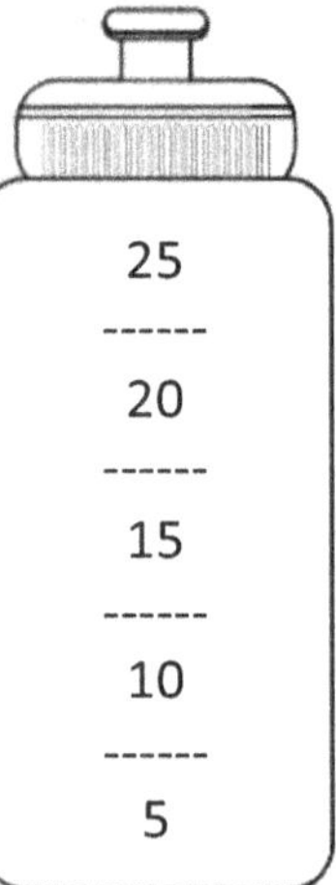

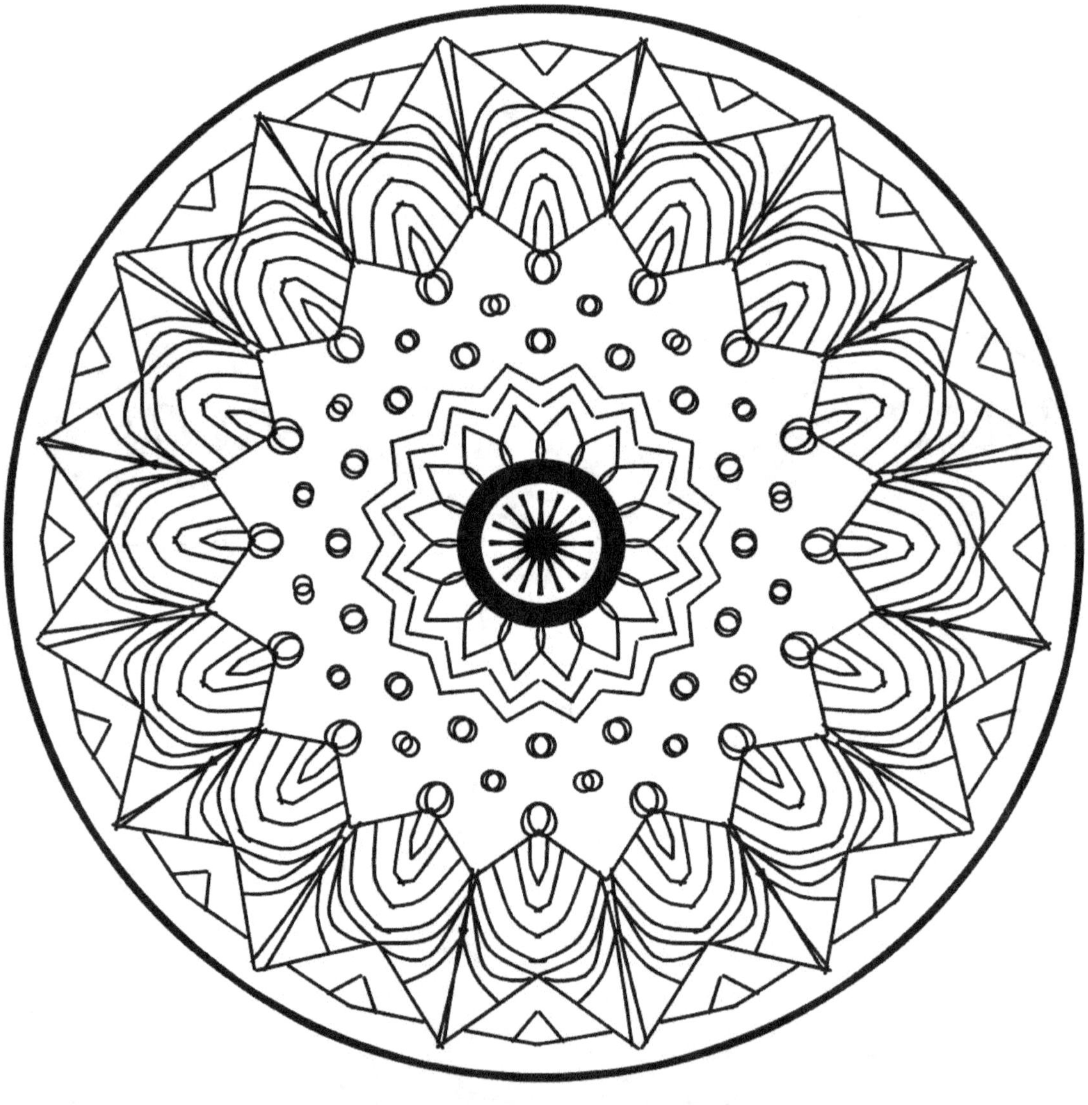

Day Twenty-eight _______

5:00 _______________________

6:00 _______________________

7:00 _______________________

8:00 _______________________

9:00 _______________________

10:00 _______________________

11:00 _______________________

Noon _______________________

1:00 _______________________

2:00 _______________________

3:00 _______________________

4:00 _______________________

5:00 _______________________

6:00 _______________________

7:00 _______________________

8:00 _______________________

9:00 _______________________

10:00 _______________________

11:00 _______________________

Midnight _______________________

____

____

____

____

____

How do identify with being
a unicorn?

____

____

____

____

____

____

The Stella Society Workout

Exercise	Set 1	Set 2	Set 3	Set 4	Set 5	notes

Time started: _____________ Time ended: _______________

Location: ____

Feelings before training: 🙂 😐 🙁 😜 😠 😟 😇 😎

Feelings after training 🙂 😐 🙁 😜 😠 😟 😇 😎

NUTRITION

Meal 1

time eaten: _________

Meal 2

time eaten: _________

Meal 3

time eaten: _________

Meal 4

time eaten: _________

Meal 5

time eaten: _________

Hydration

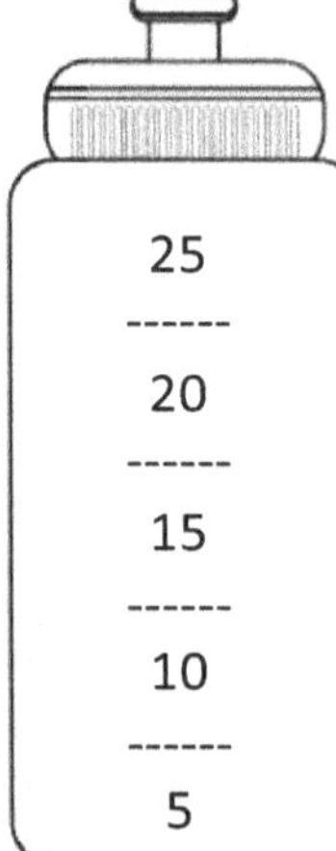

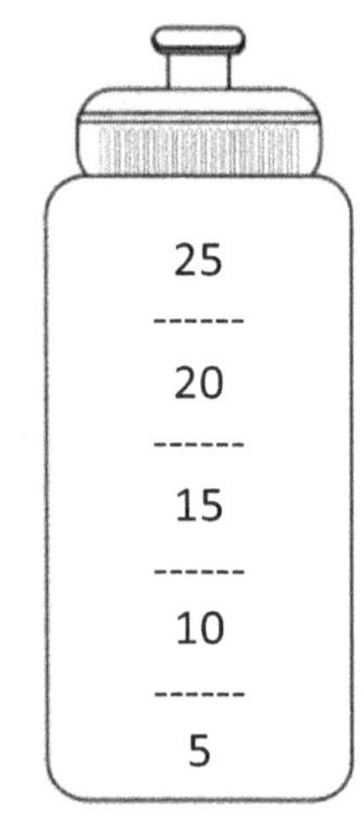

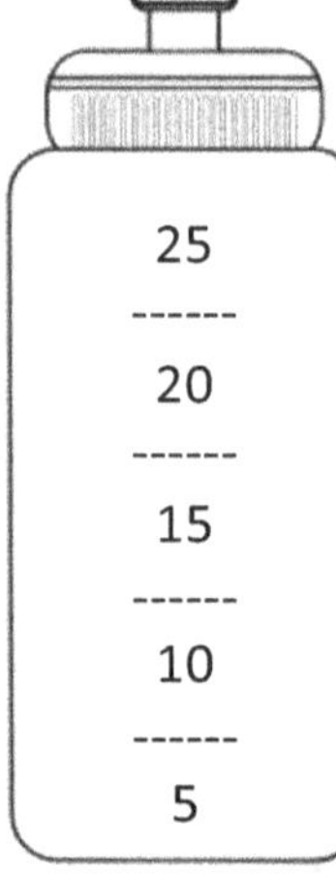

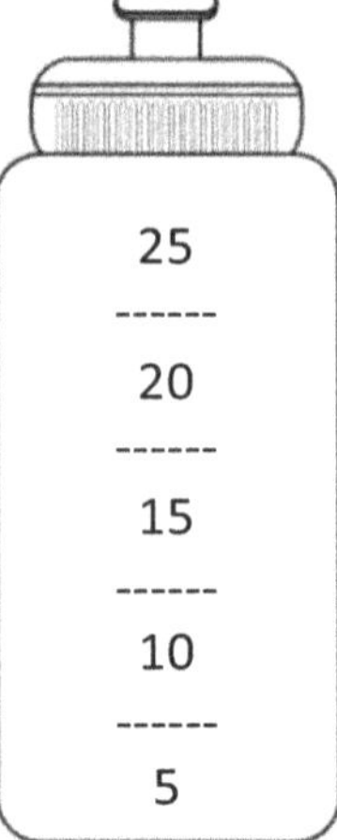

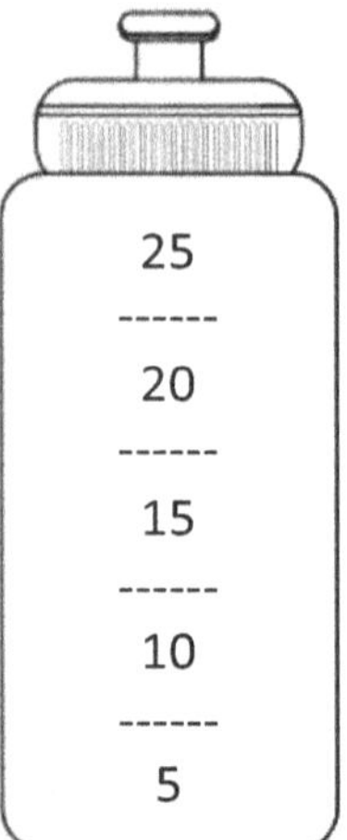

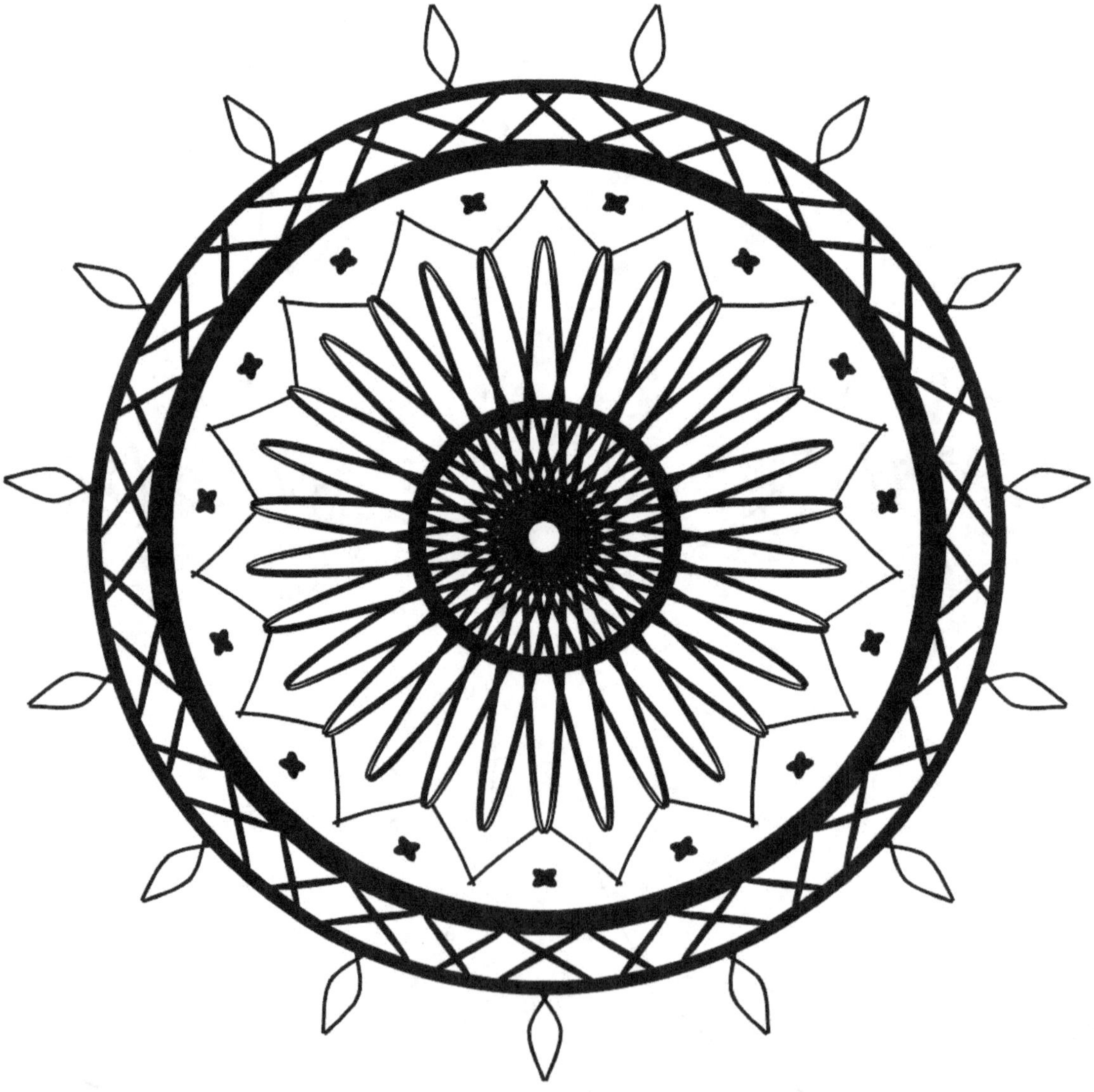

Day Twenty-nine _______

5:00 ______________________

6:00 ______________________

7:00 ______________________

8:00 ______________________

9:00 ______________________

10:00 ______________________

11:00 ______________________

Noon ______________________

1:00 ______________________

2:00 ______________________

3:00 ______________________

4:00 ______________________

5:00 ______________________

6:00 ______________________

7:00 ______________________

8:00 ______________________

9:00 ______________________

10:00 ______________________

11:00 ______________________

Midnight ______________________

top priorities for today

Today's victories

You have permission to be a savage. What do you do with it?

The Stella Society Workout

Exercise	Set 1	Set 2	Set 3	Set 4	Set 5	notes

Time started: _____________ Time ended: _____________

Location: ____

Feelings before training:

Feelings after training

NUTRITION

Meal 1

time eaten: _________

Meal 2

time eaten: _________

Meal 3

time eaten: _________

Meal 4

time eaten: _________

Meal 5

time eaten: _________

Hydration

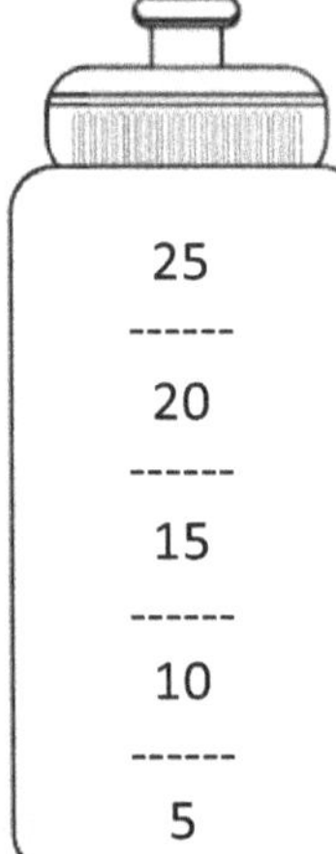

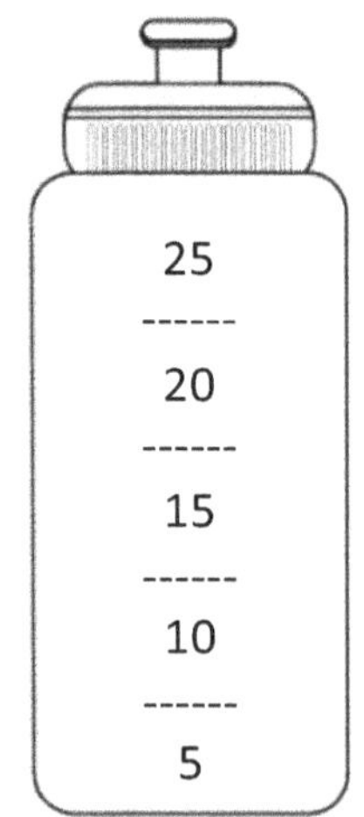

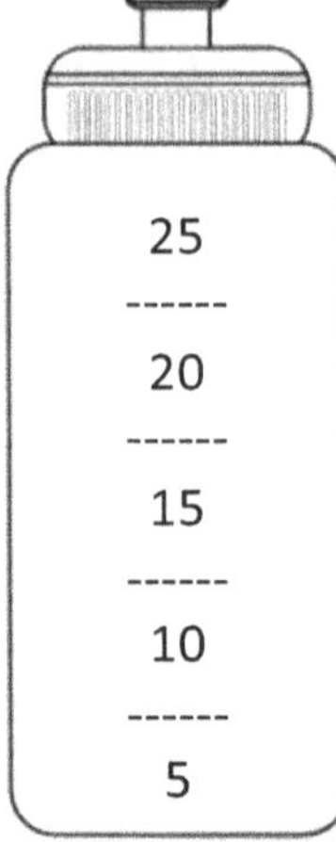

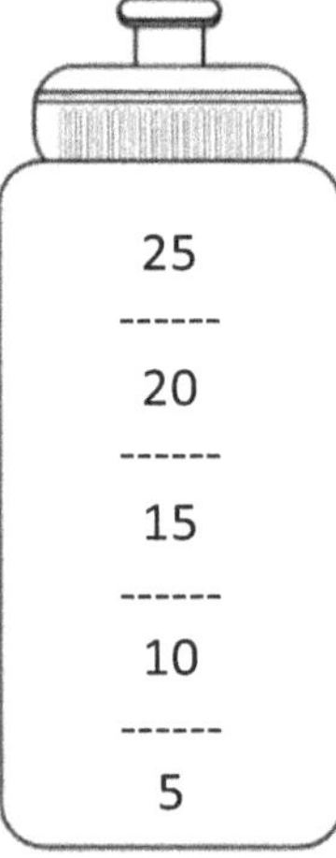

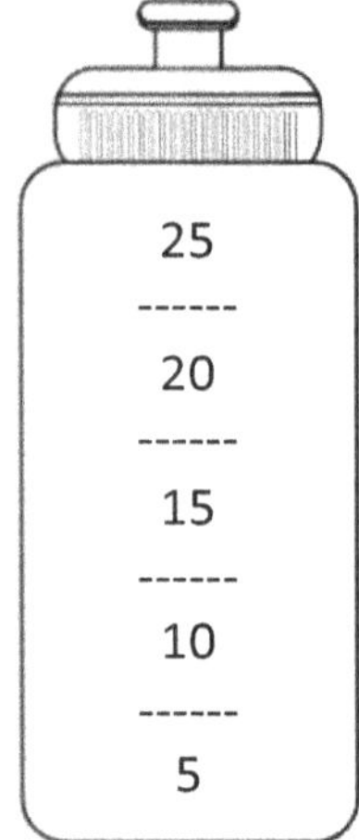

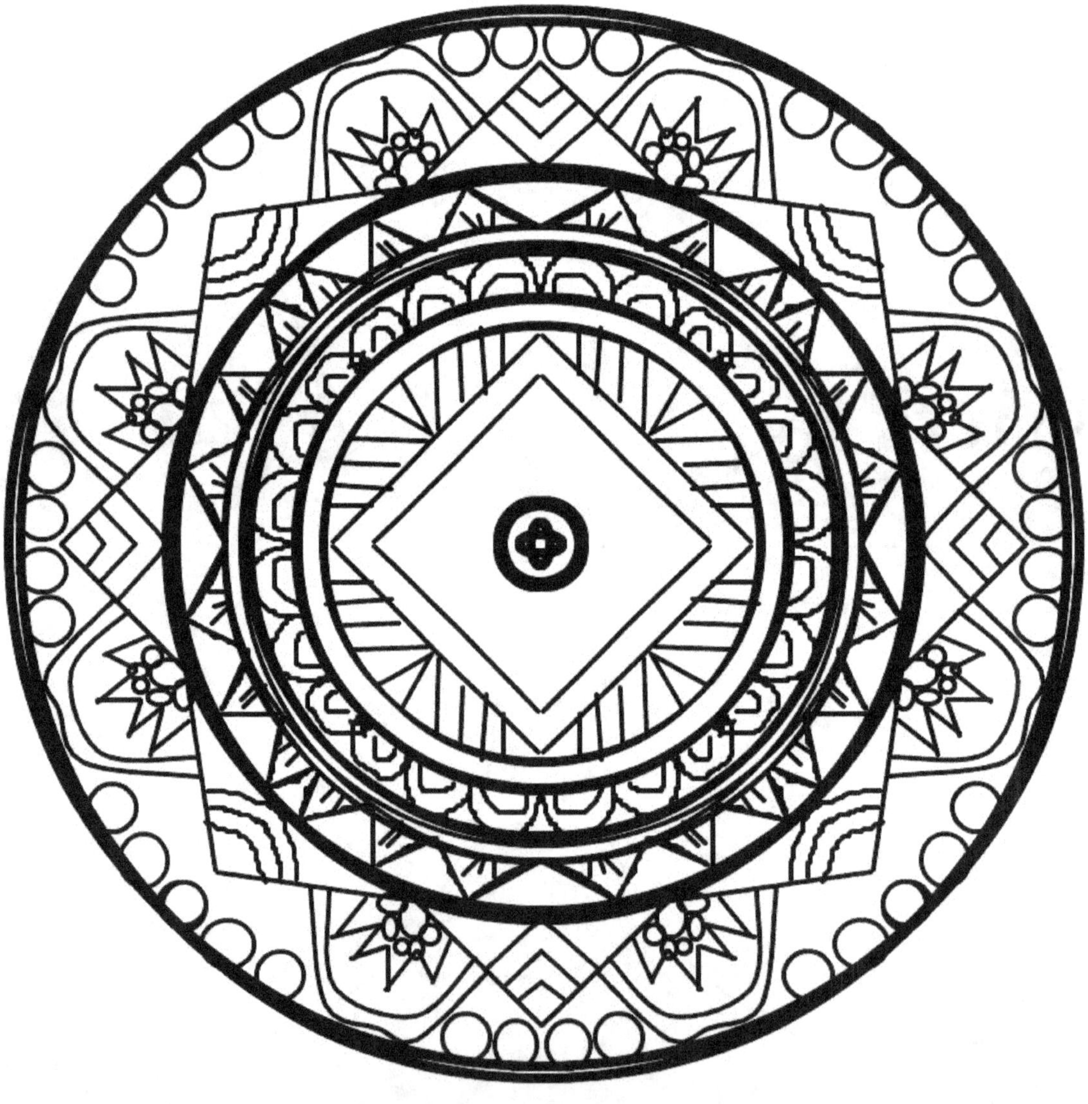

Measurements

P R O G R E S S

DATE: __________

Weight: ______

Neck ______

Shoulders ______

Chest ______

Bicep / upper arm left ________ right ______

Forearm left ________ right ______

Waist ______

Hips ______

Thighs left ________ right ______

Calf left ________ right ______

C H E C K

It's Not A Diet,
It's A Lifestyle Change

Day Thirty ______

5:00 ______________________

6:00 ______________________

7:00 ______________________

8:00 ______________________

9:00 ______________________

10:00 ______________________

11:00 ______________________

Noon ______________________

1:00 ______________________

2:00 ______________________

3:00 ______________________

4:00 ______________________

5:00 ______________________

6:00 ______________________

7:00 ______________________

8:00 ______________________

9:00 ______________________

10:00 ______________________

11:00 ______________________

Midnight ______________________

How can you be powerful and
sensitive at the same time?

The Stella Society Workout

Exercise	Set 1	Set 2	Set 3	Set 4	Set 5	notes

Time started: _____________ Time ended: _____________

Location: ____

Feelings before training:

Feelings after training

NUTRITION

Meal 1

time eaten: _________

Meal 2

time eaten: _________

Meal 3

time eaten: _________

Meal 4

time eaten: _________

Meal 5

time eaten: _________

Hydration

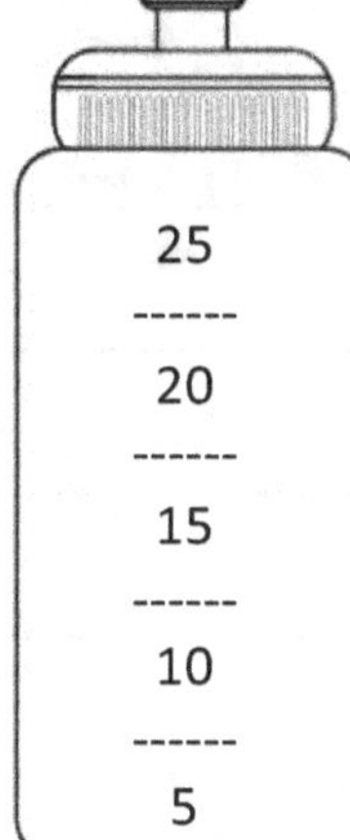

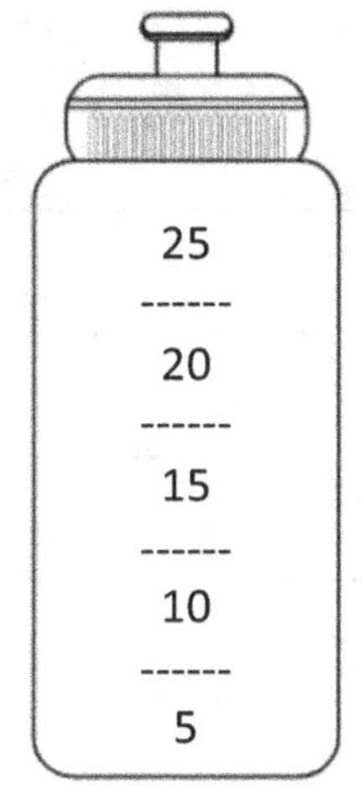

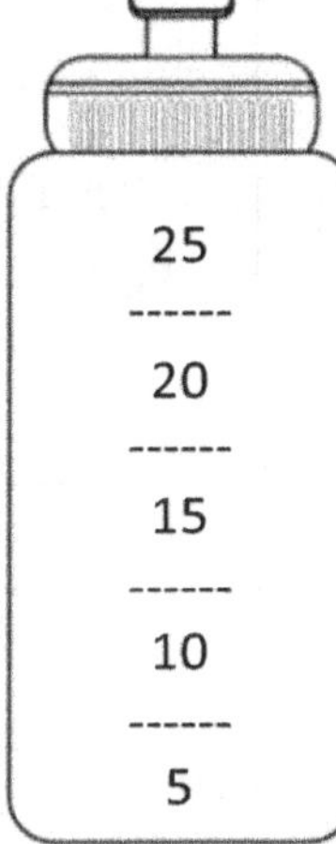

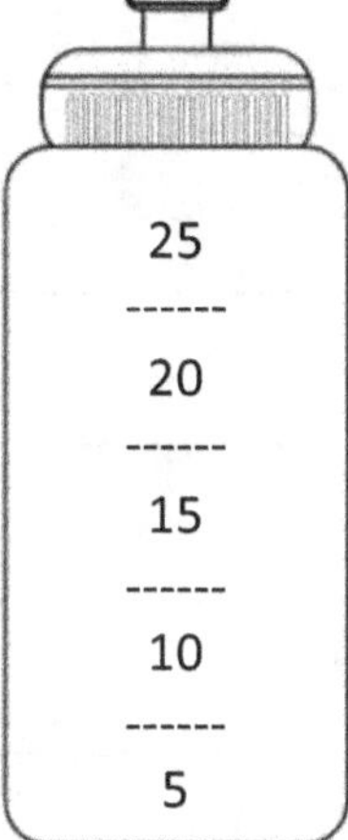

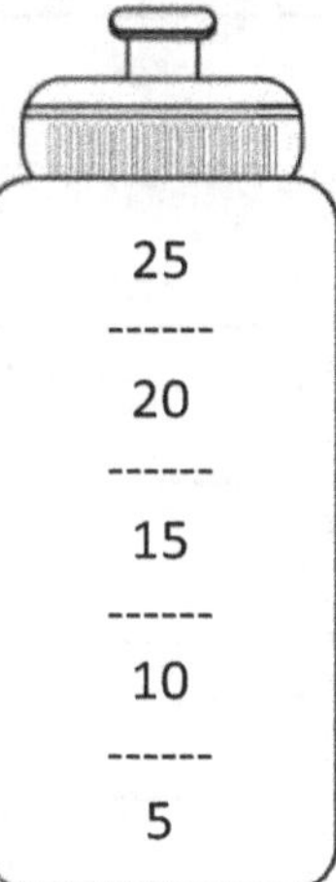

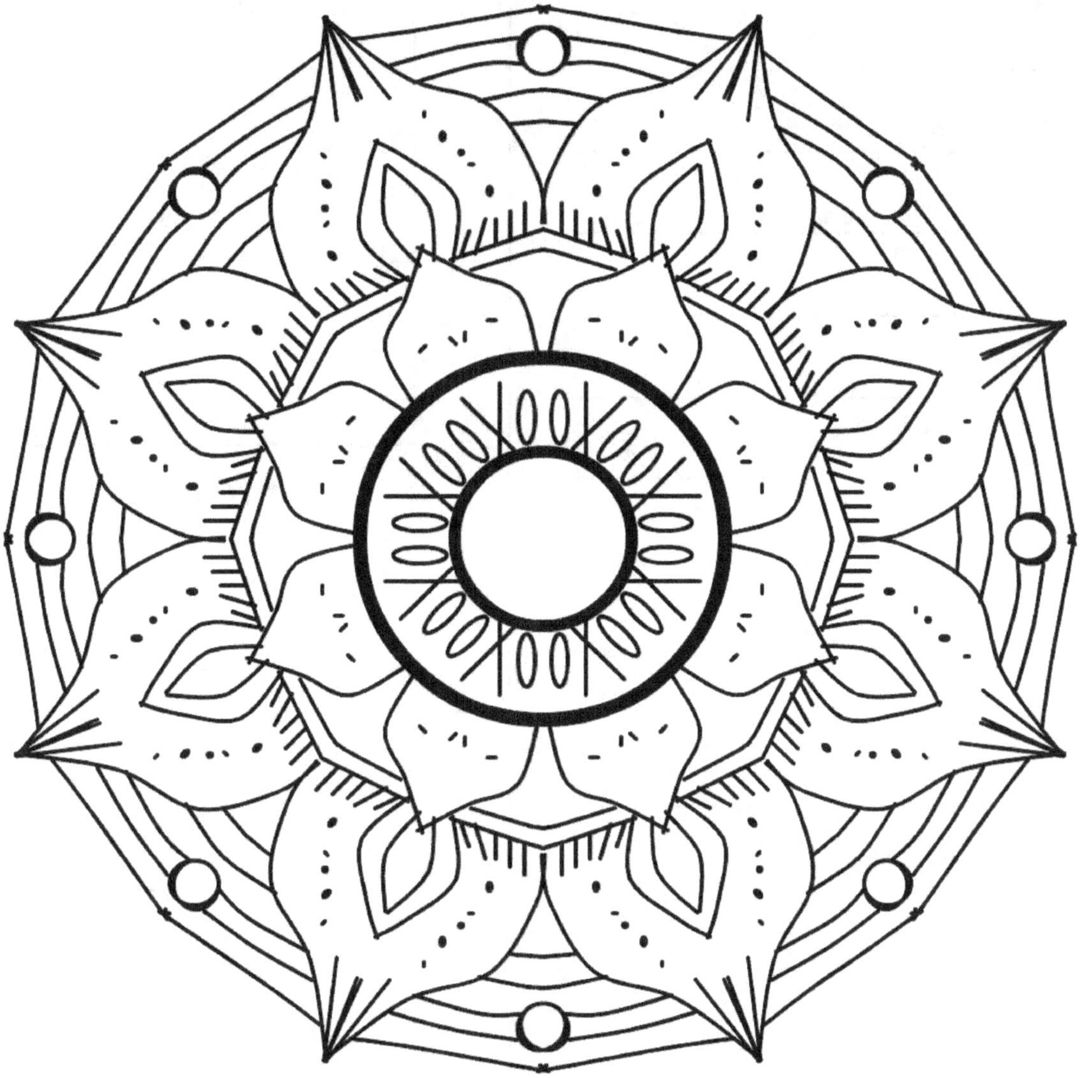

Day Thirty-one _______

5:00 _______________________

6:00 _______________________

7:00 _______________________

8:00 _______________________

9:00 _______________________

10:00 _______________________

11:00 _______________________

Noon _______________________

1:00 _______________________

2:00 _______________________

3:00 _______________________

4:00 _______________________

5:00 _______________________

6:00 _______________________

7:00 _______________________

8:00 _______________________

9:00 _______________________

10:00 _______________________

11:00 _______________________

Midnight _______________________

top priorities for today 🎯

____

____

____

____

Today's victories 🏆

Is being forceful a bad thing?

____

____

____

____

____

____

The Stella Society Workout

Exercise	Set 1	Set 2	Set 3	Set 4	Set 5	notes

Time started: _____________ Time ended: _____________

Location: _______________________________________

Feelings before training: 🙂 😐 🙁 😜 😠 😟 😇 😎

Feelings after training 🙂 😐 🙁 😜 😠 😟 😇 😎

NUTRITION

Meal 1

time eaten: _________

Meal 2

time eaten: _________

Meal 3

time eaten: _________

Meal 4

time eaten: _________

Meal 5

time eaten: _________

Hydration

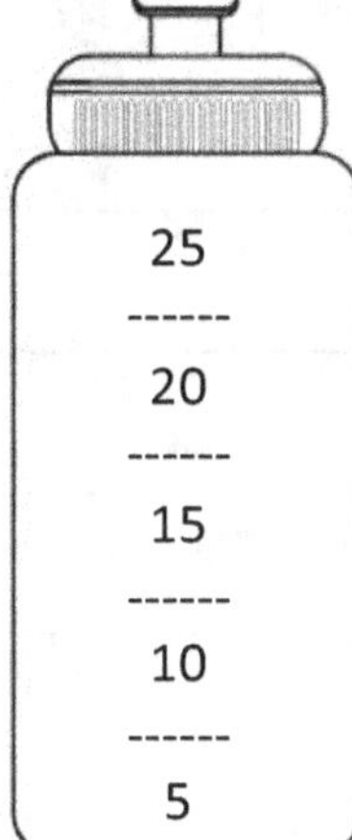

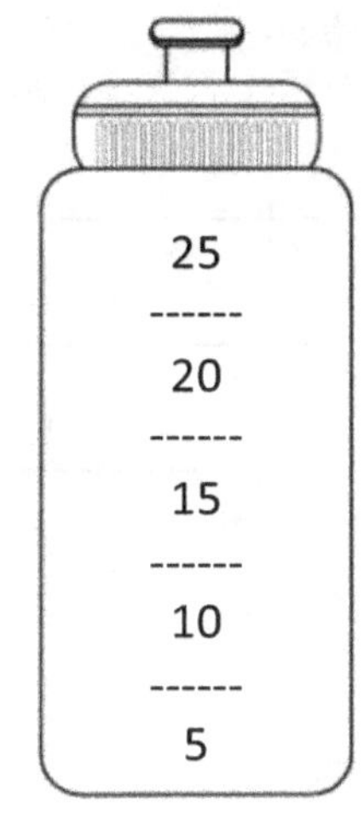

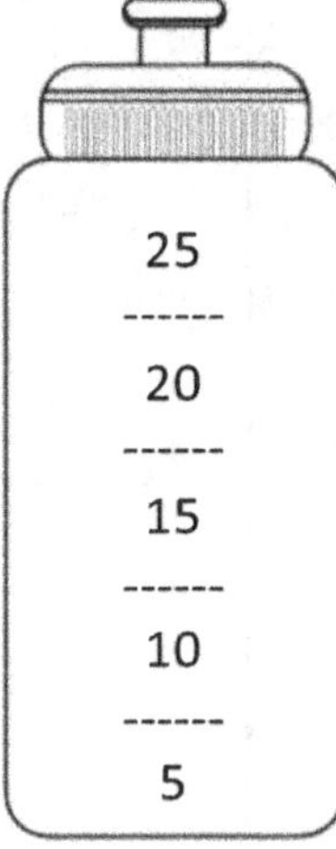

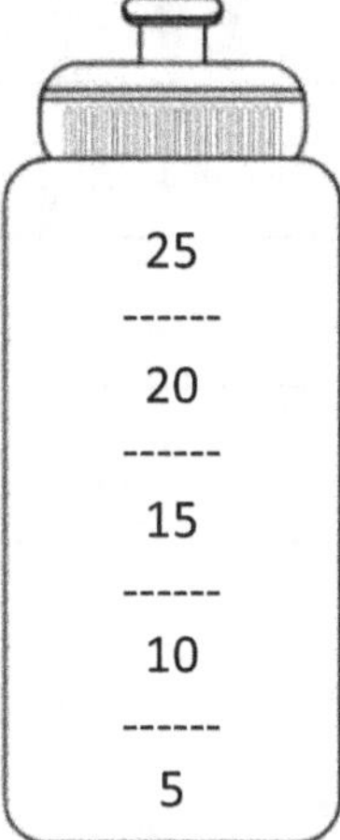

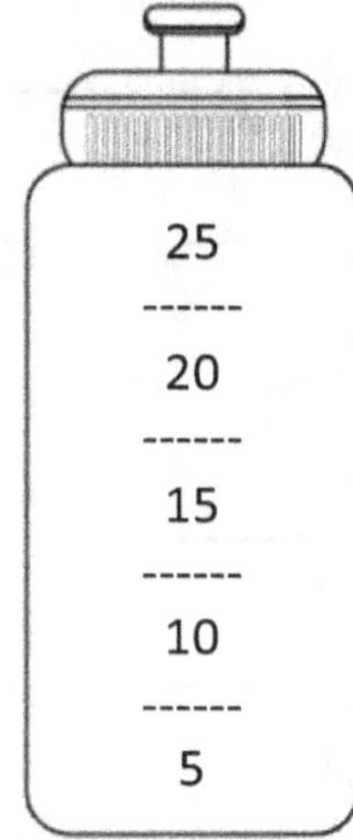

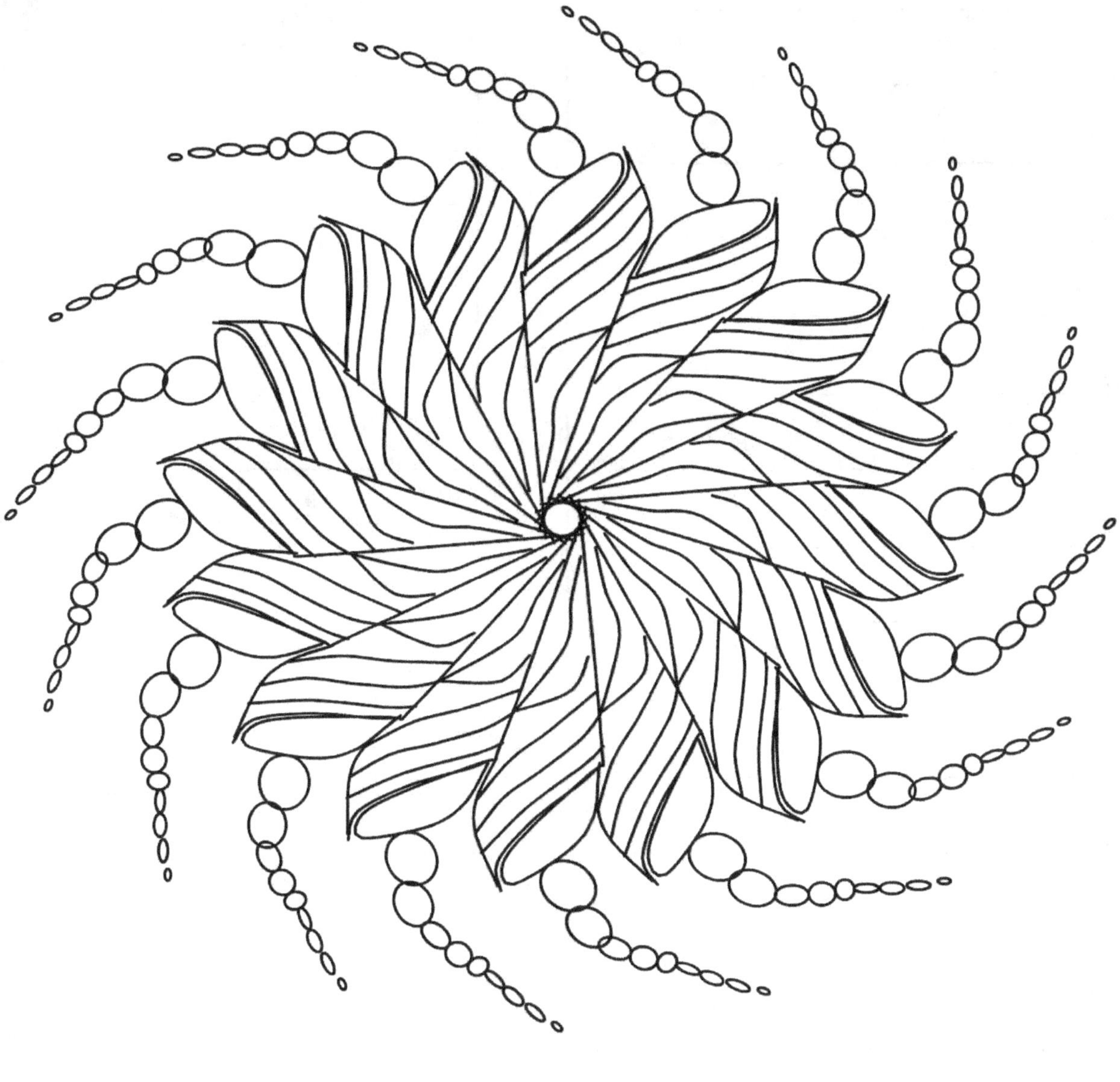

Day Thirty-two _______

5:00 ________________	

5:00 ___________________

6:00 ___________________

7:00 ___________________

8:00 ___________________

9:00 ___________________

10:00 __________________

11:00 __________________

Noon ___________________

1:00 ___________________

2:00 ___________________

3:00 ___________________

4:00 ___________________

5:00 ___________________

6:00 ___________________

7:00 ___________________

8:00 ___________________

9:00 ___________________

10:00 __________________

11:00 __________________

Midnight _______________

The Stella Society Workout

Exercise	Set 1	Set 2	Set 3	Set 4	Set 5	notes

Time started: _____________ Time ended: _____________

Location: _______________________________________

Feelings before training:

Feelings after training

NUTRITION

Meal 1
time eaten: _________

Meal 2
time eaten: _________

Meal 3
time eaten: _________

Meal 4
time eaten: _________

Meal 5
time eaten: _________

Hydration

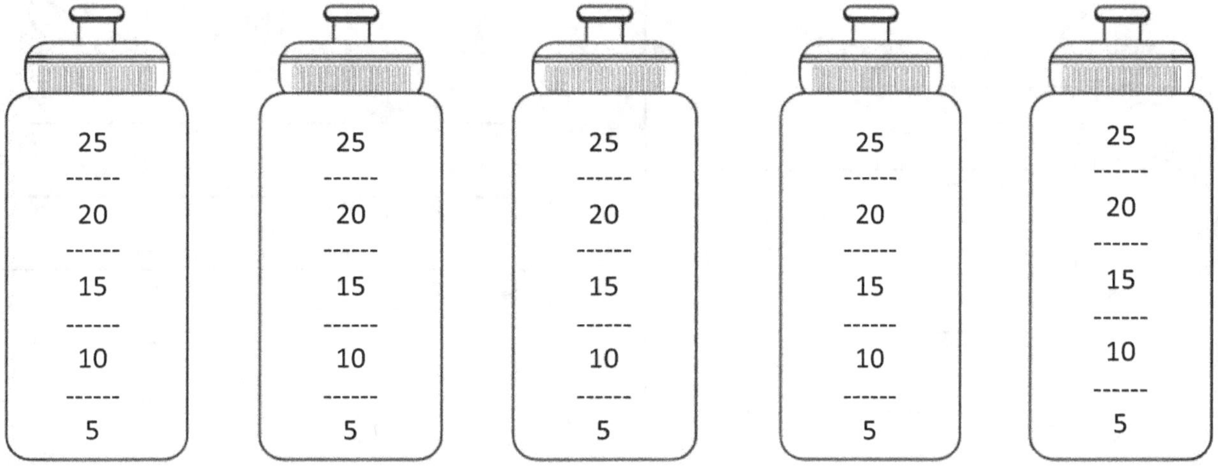

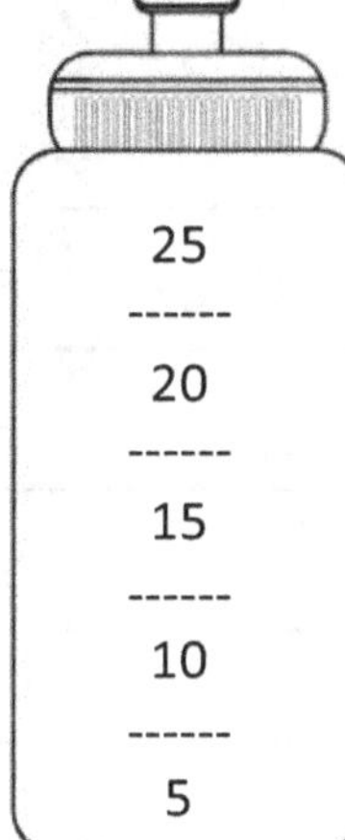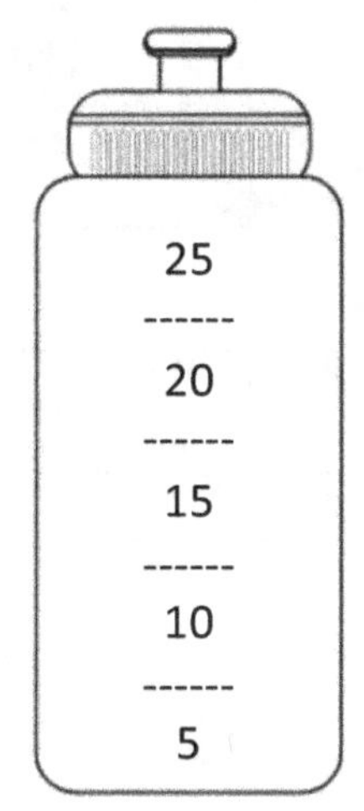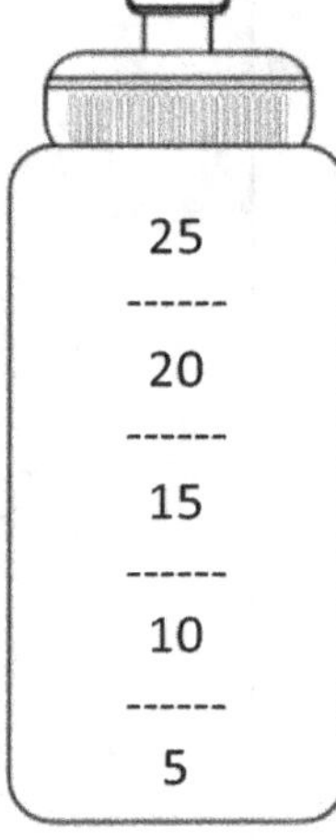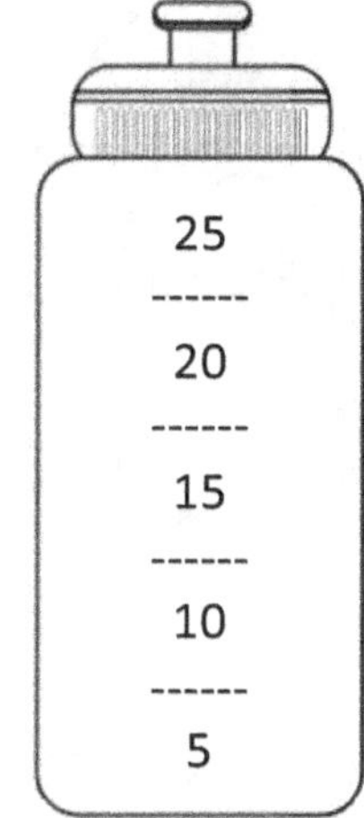

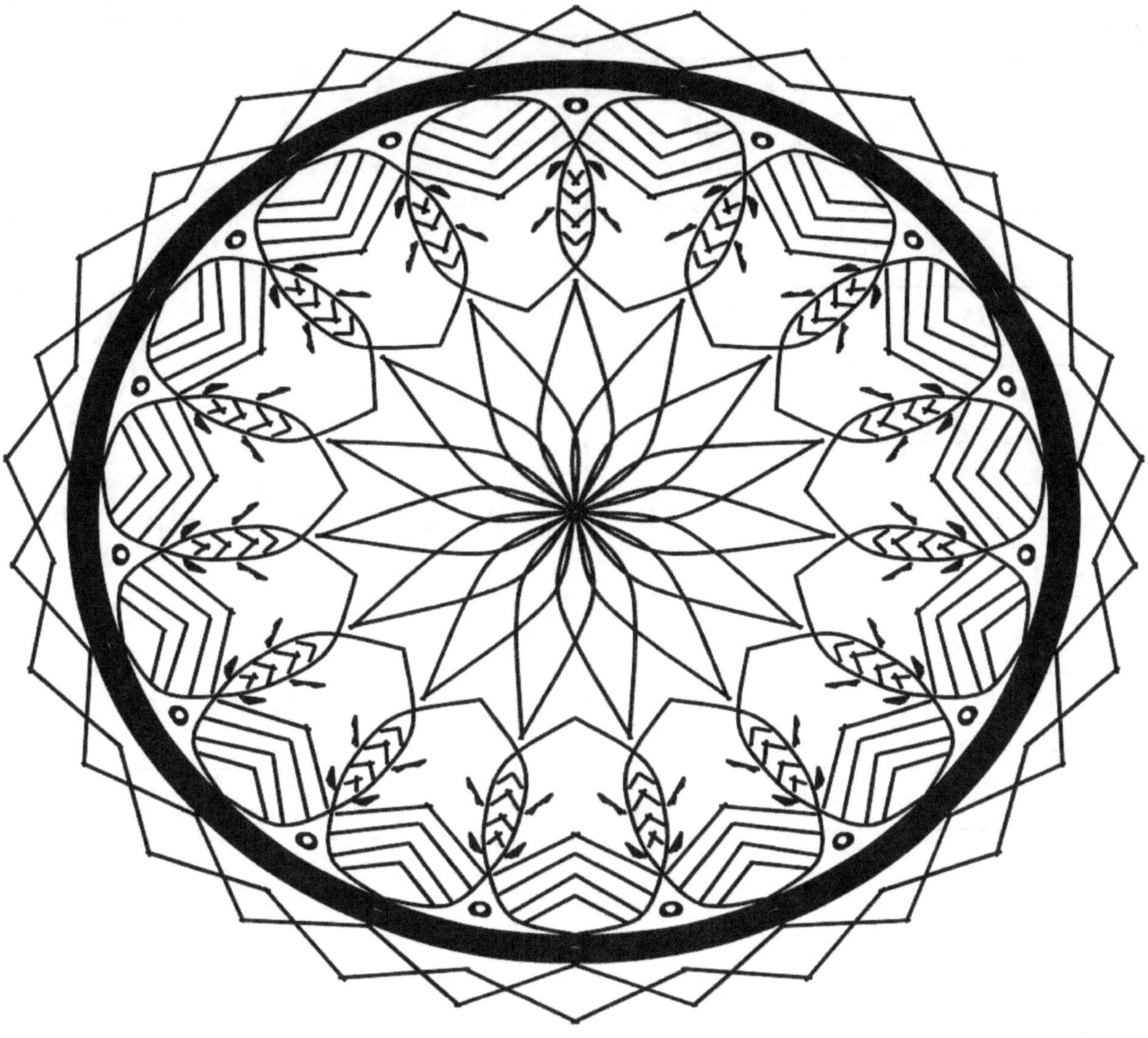

Day Thirty-three _______

5:00 _______________________

6:00 _______________________

7:00 _______________________

8:00 _______________________

9:00 _______________________

10:00 ______________________

11:00 ______________________

Noon _______________________

1:00 _______________________

2:00 _______________________

3:00 _______________________

4:00 _______________________

5:00 _______________________

6:00 _______________________

7:00 _______________________

8:00 _______________________

9:00 _______________________

10:00 ______________________

11:00 ______________________

Midnight ___________________

top priorities for today

____

____

____

____

Today's victories

How are you glowing today?

____

____

____

____

____

____

The Stella Society Workout

Exercise	Set 1	Set 2	Set 3	Set 4	Set 5	notes

Time started: _____________ Time ended: _____________

Location: ____

Feelings before training:

Feelings after training

NUTRITION

Meal 1
time eaten: _________

Meal 2
time eaten: _________

Meal 3
time eaten: _________

Meal 4
time eaten: _________

Meal 5
time eaten: _________

Hydration

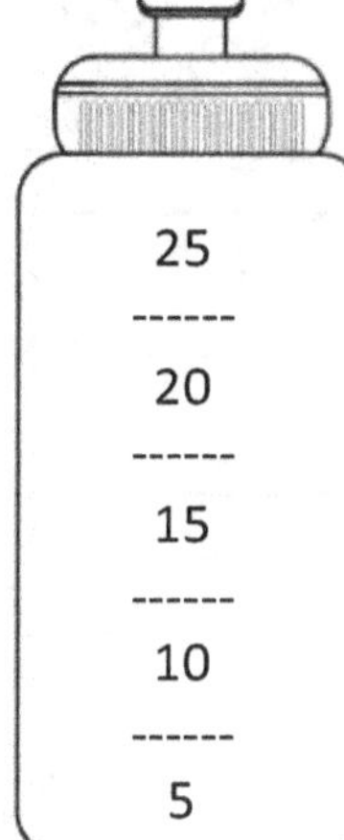
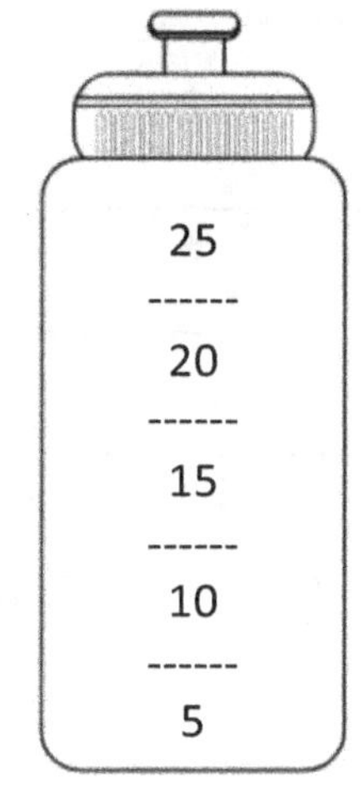
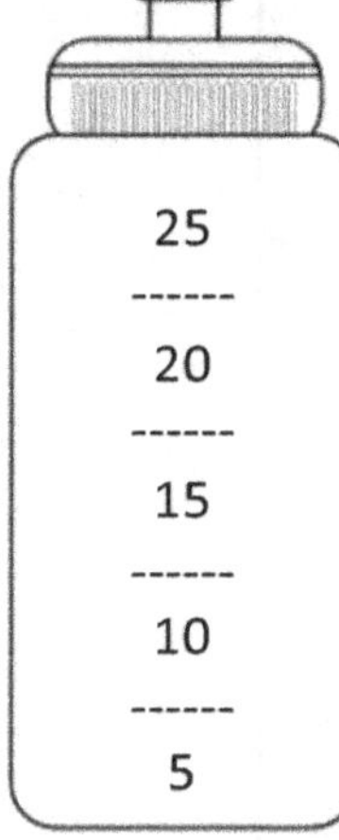
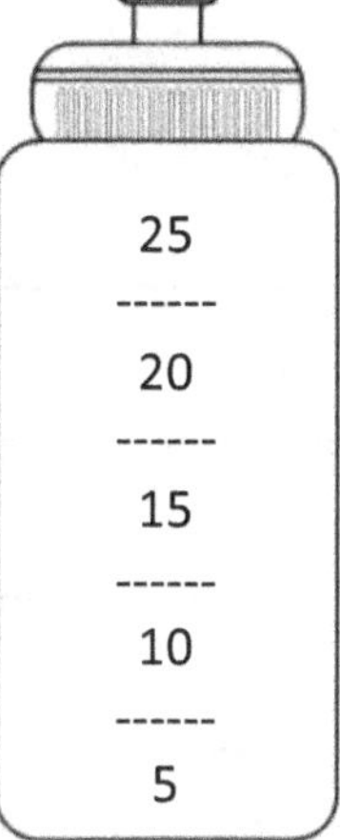
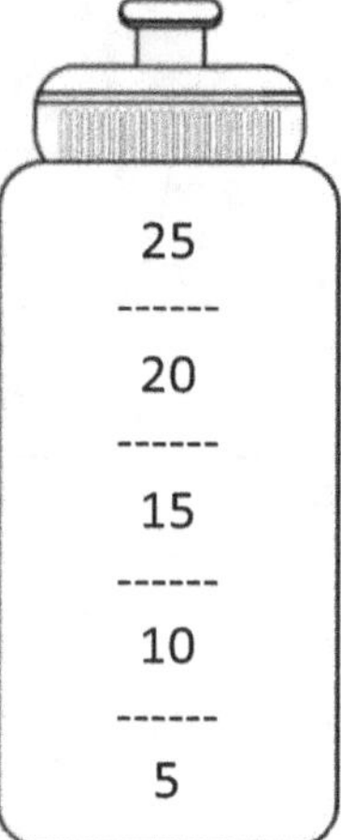

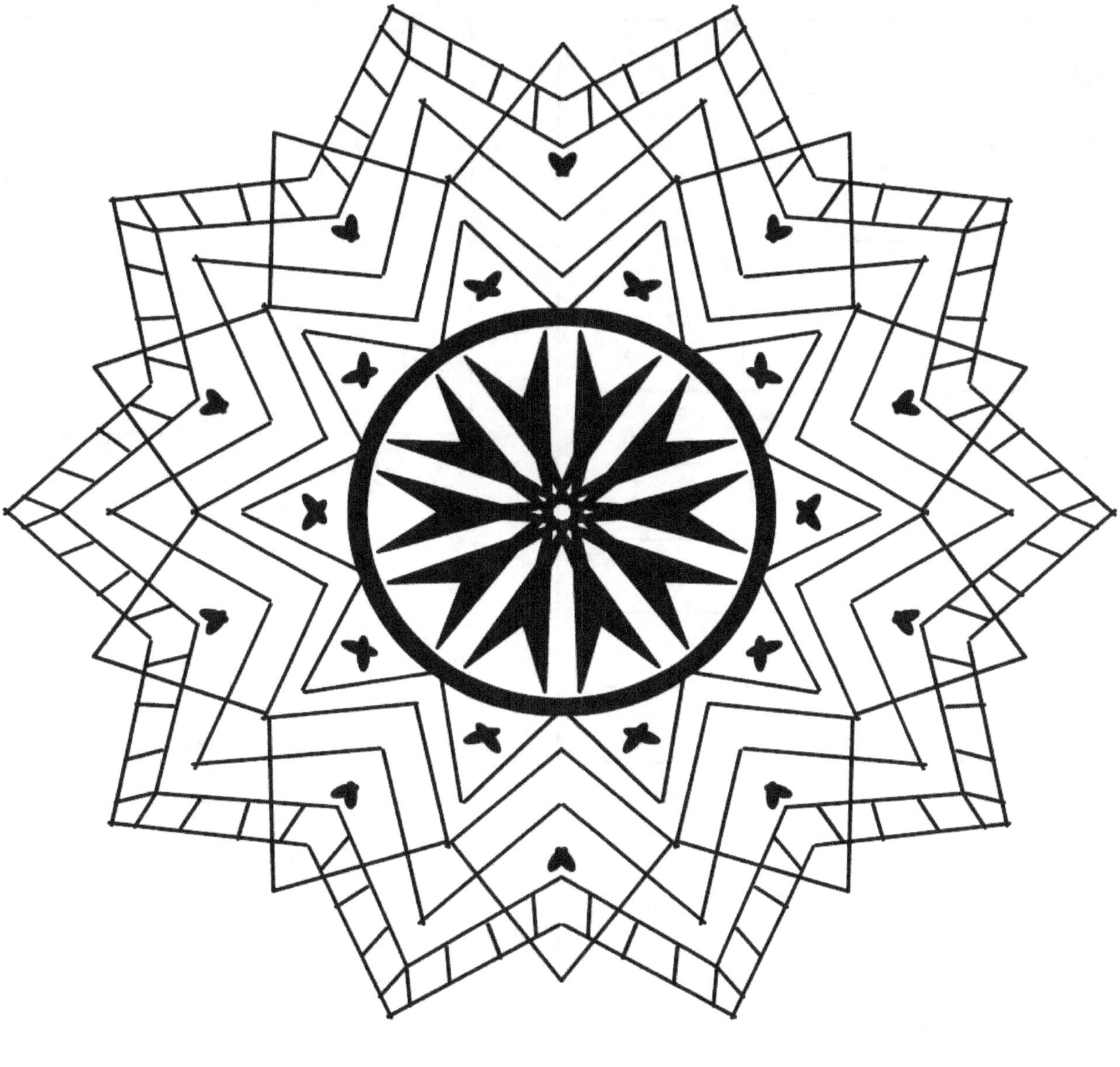

Day Thirty-four ______

5:00 _________________	

5:00 ____________________
6:00 ____________________
7:00 ____________________
8:00 ____________________
9:00 ____________________
10:00 __________________
11:00 __________________
Noon ___________________
1:00 ____________________
2:00 ____________________
3:00 ____________________
4:00 ____________________
5:00 ____________________
6:00 ____________________
7:00 ____________________
8:00 ____________________
9:00 ____________________
10:00 __________________
11:00 __________________
Midnight _______________

top priorities for today

Today's victories

What are you dedicated to
do at this moment?

The Stella Society Workout

Exercise	Set 1	Set 2	Set 3	Set 4	Set 5	notes

Time started: _____________ Time ended: _____________

Location: ____

Feelings before training: 😊 😐 ☹️ 😜 😠 😕 😇 😎

Feelings after training 😊 😐 ☹️ 😜 😠 😕 😇 😎

NUTRITION

Meal 1
time eaten: _________

Meal 2
time eaten: _________

Meal 3
time eaten: _________

Meal 4
time eaten: _________

Meal 5
time eaten: _________

Hydration

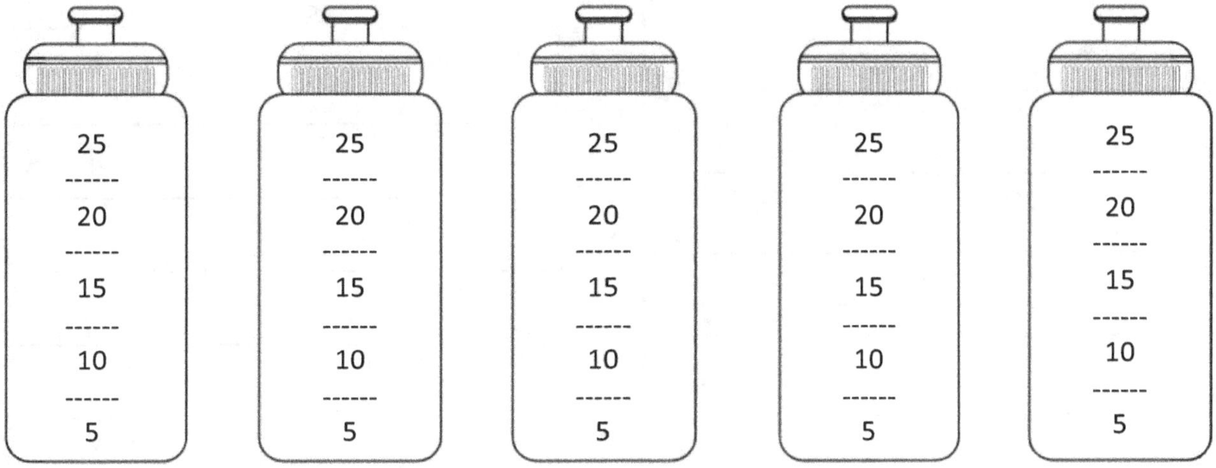

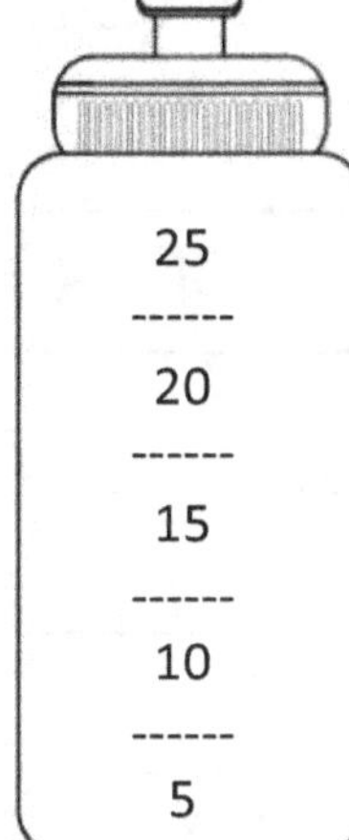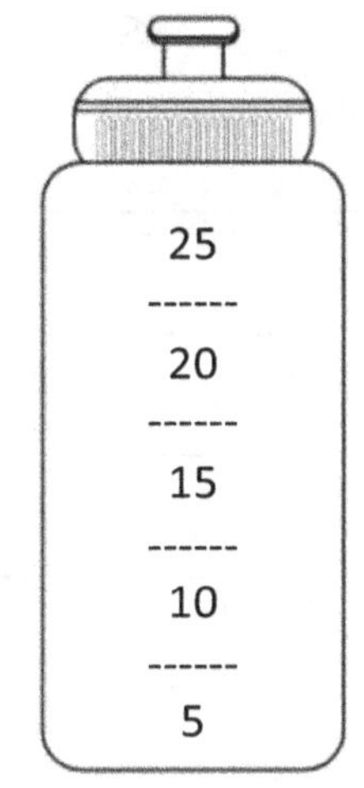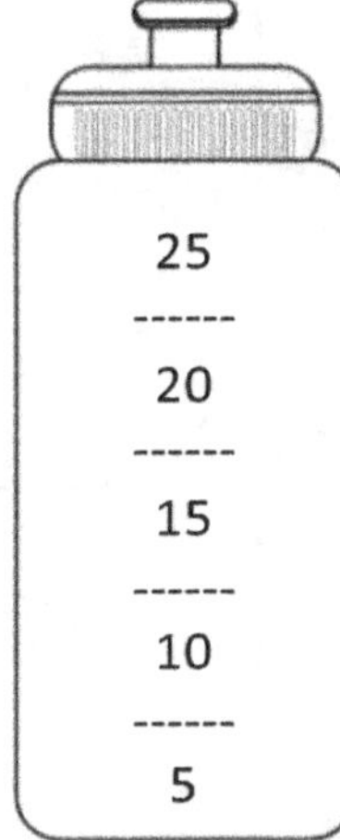

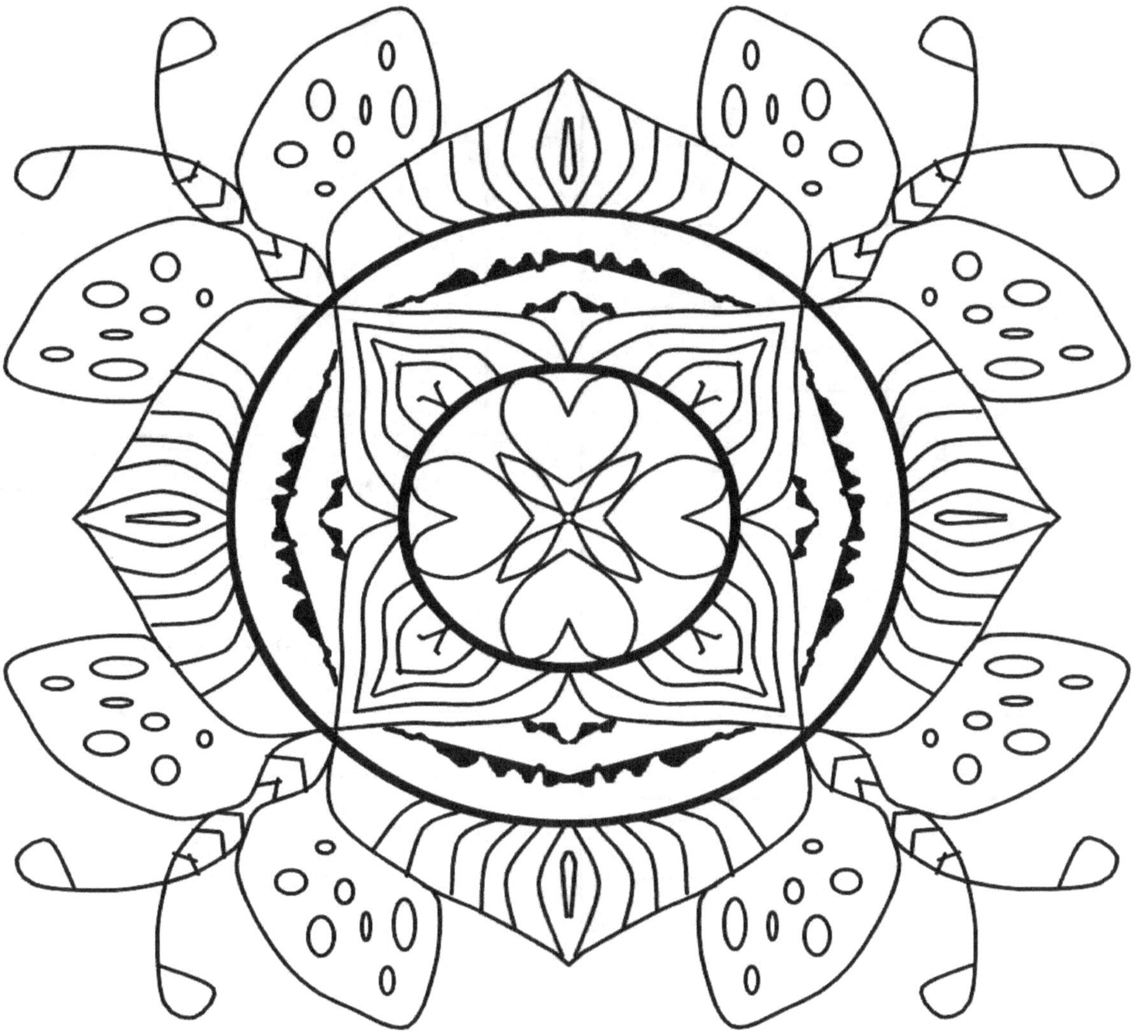

Day Thirty-five _______

5:00 _______________________

6:00 _______________________

7:00 _______________________

8:00 _______________________

9:00 _______________________

10:00 _______________________

11:00 _______________________

Noon _______________________

1:00 _______________________

2:00 _______________________

3:00 _______________________

4:00 _______________________

5:00 _______________________

6:00 _______________________

7:00 _______________________

8:00 _______________________

9:00 _______________________

10:00 _______________________

11:00 _______________________

Midnight _______________________

top priorities for today 🎯

____
____
____
____
____

Today's victories 🏆

Who is more determined
than you?

____
____
____
____
____
____

The *Stella Society* Workout

Exercise	Set 1	Set 2	Set 3	Set 4	Set 5	notes

Time started: _____________ Time ended: _____________

Location: ____

Feelings before training: 🙂 😑 🙁 😜 😠 😕 😇 😎

Feelings after training 🙂 😑 🙁 😜 😠 😕 😇 😎

NUTRITION

Meal 1
time eaten: _________

Meal 2
time eaten: _________

Meal 3
time eaten: _________

Meal 4
time eaten: _________

Meal 5
time eaten: _________

Hydration

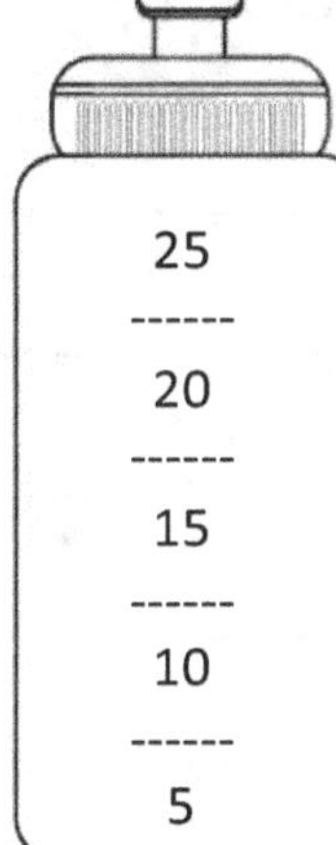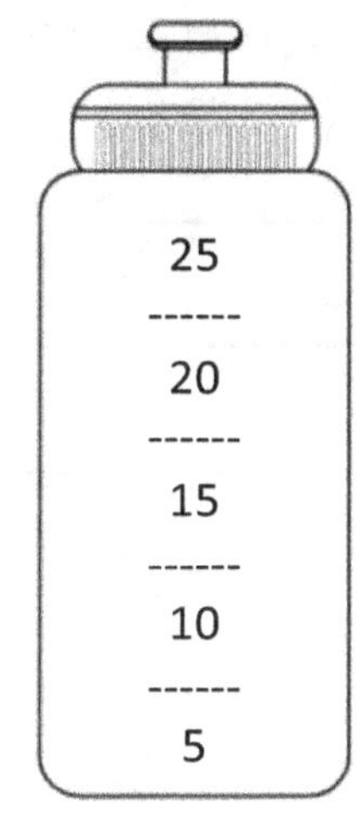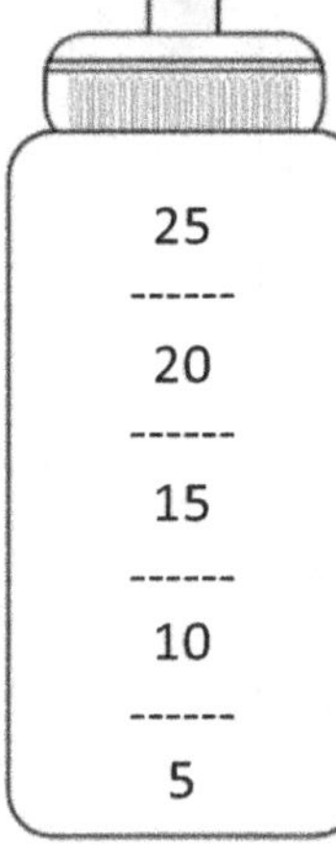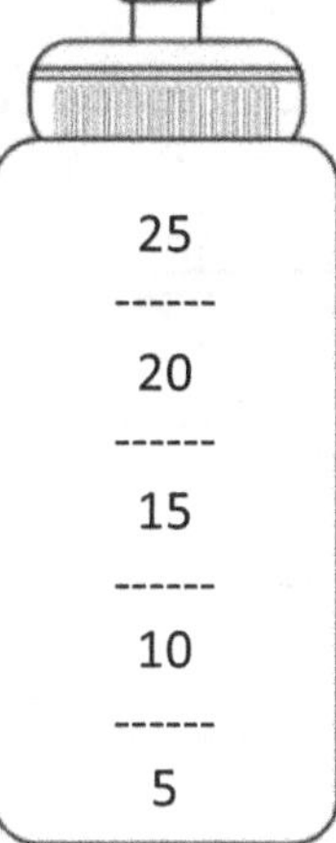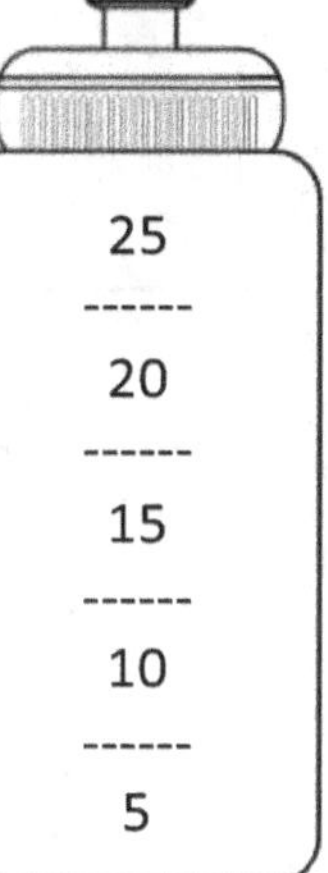

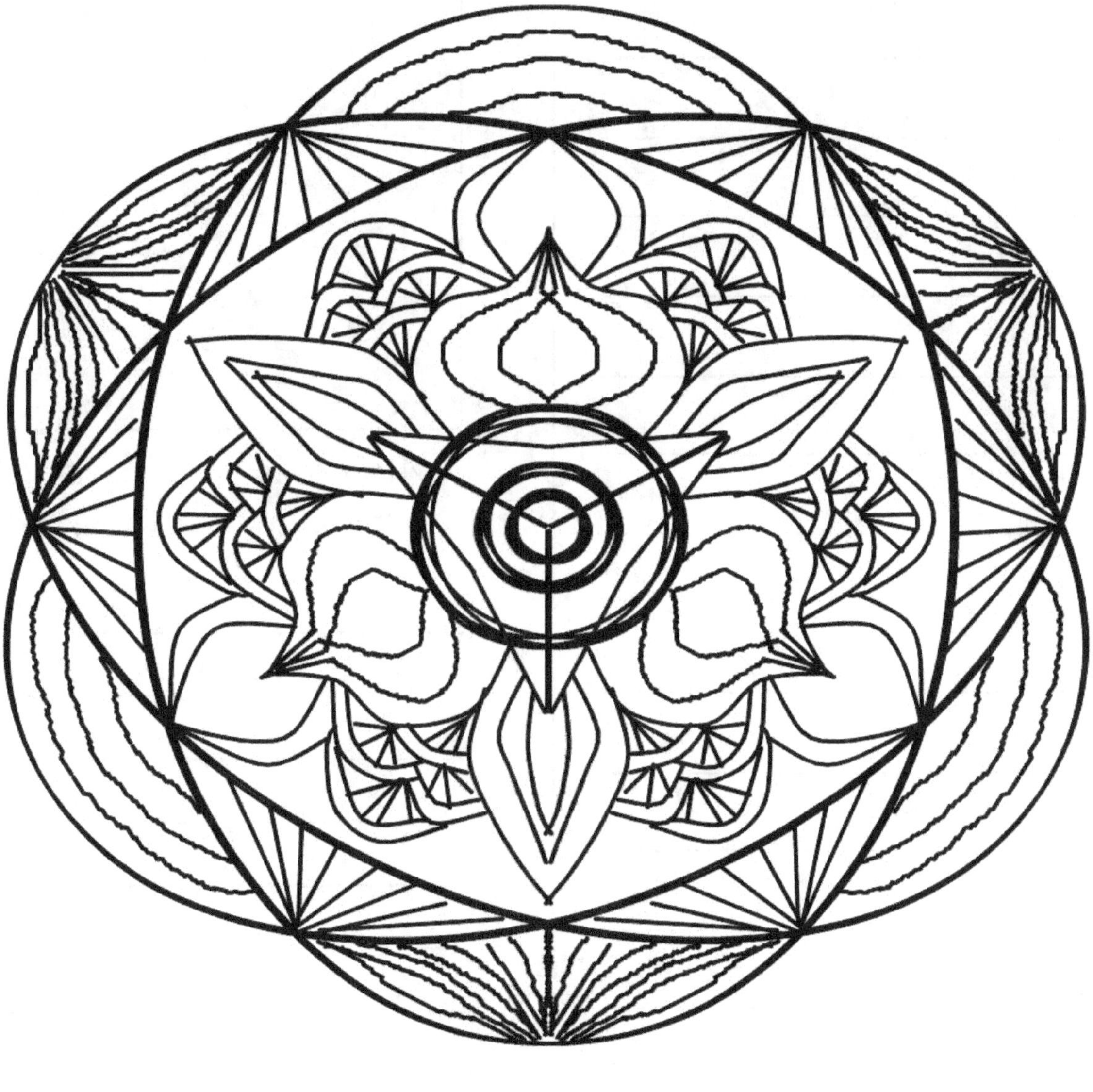

Day Thirty-six ______

5:00 ______________________

6:00 ______________________

7:00 ______________________

8:00 ______________________

9:00 ______________________

10:00 ______________________

11:00 ______________________

Noon ______________________

1:00 ______________________

2:00 ______________________

3:00 ______________________

4:00 ______________________

5:00 ______________________

6:00 ______________________

7:00 ______________________

8:00 ______________________

9:00 ______________________

10:00 ______________________

11:00 ______________________

Midnight __________________

top priorities for today

Today's victories

Who needs your acceptance
of change and why?

The *Stella Society* Workout

Exercise	Set 1	Set 2	Set 3	Set 4	Set 5	notes

Time started: _____________ Time ended: _____________

Location: ____

Feelings before training:

Feelings after training

NUTRITION

Meal 1
time eaten: _________

Meal 2
time eaten: _________

Meal 3
time eaten: _________

Meal 4
time eaten: _________

Meal 5
time eaten: _________

Hydration

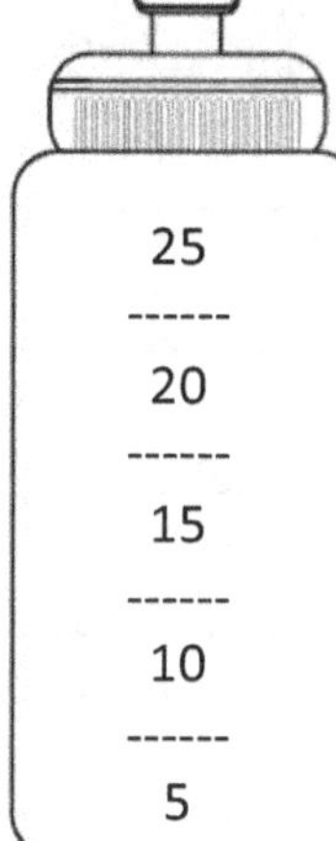

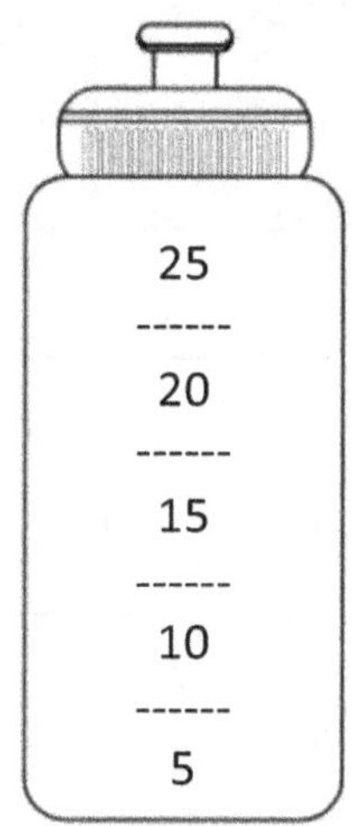

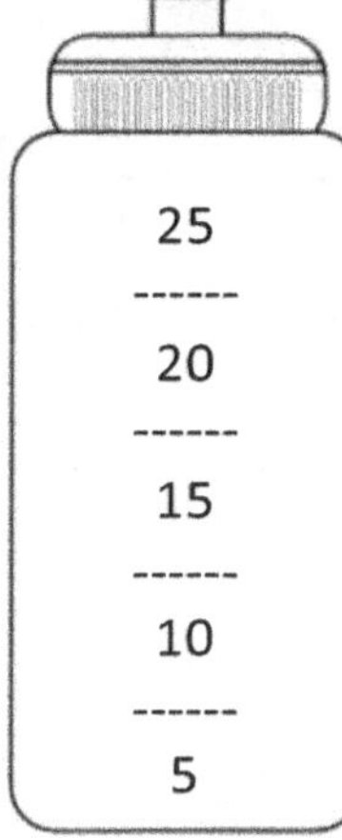

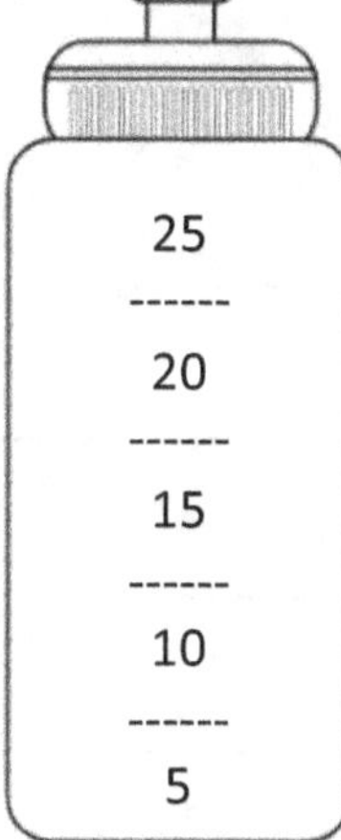

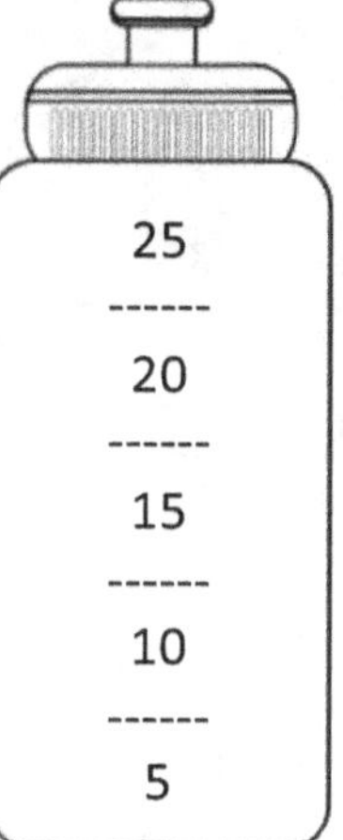

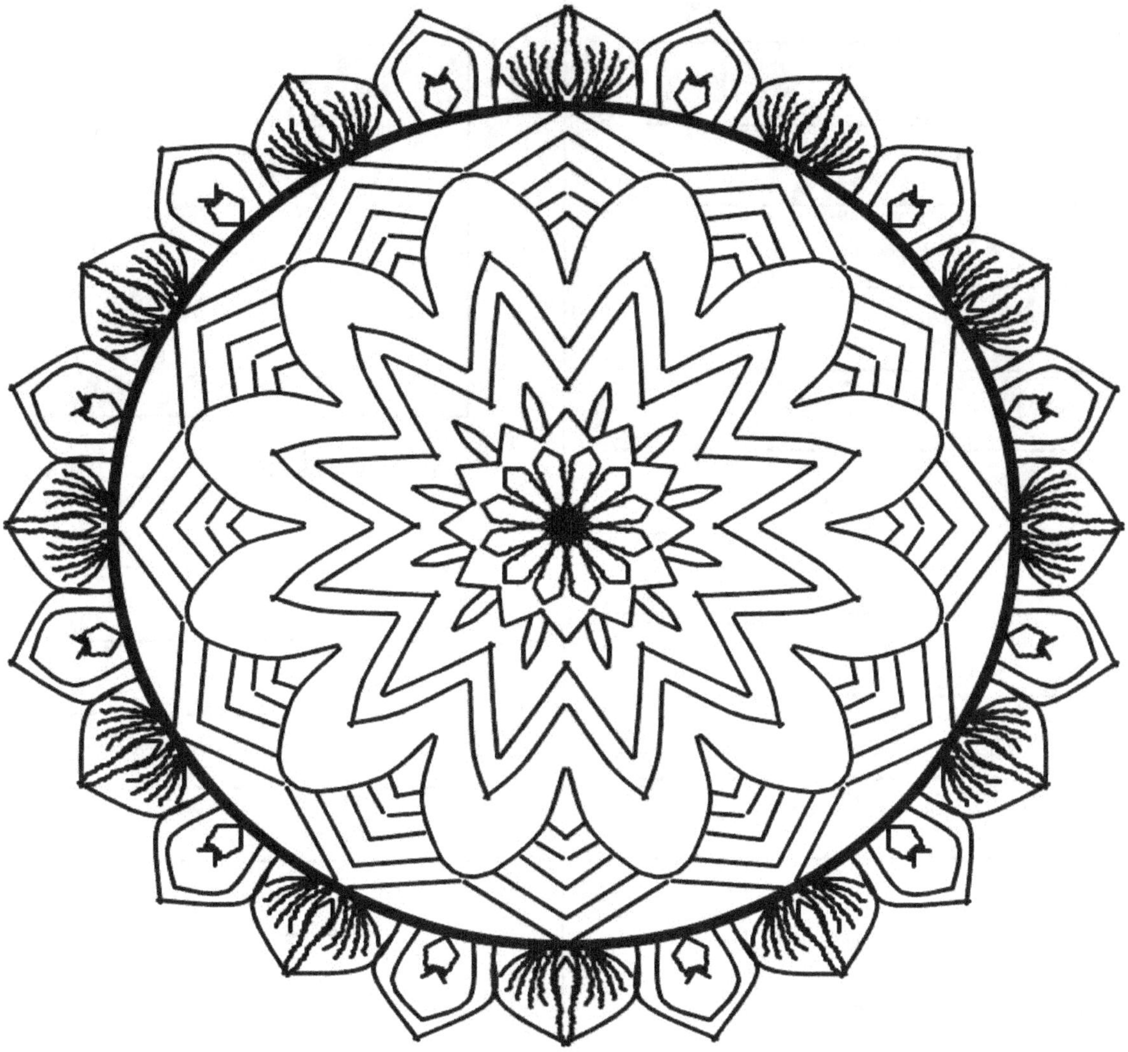

Day Thirty-seven _______

5:00 _______________________

6:00 _______________________

7:00 _______________________

8:00 _______________________

9:00 _______________________

10:00 ______________________

11:00 ______________________

Noon _______________________

1:00 _______________________

2:00 _______________________

3:00 _______________________

4:00 _______________________

5:00 _______________________

6:00 _______________________

7:00 _______________________

8:00 _______________________

9:00 _______________________

10:00 ______________________

11:00 ______________________

Midnight ____________________

Today's victories

How will you be captivating?

The Stella Society Workout

Exercise	Set 1	Set 2	Set 3	Set 4	Set 5	notes

Time started: _____________ Time ended: _______________

Location: ____

Feelings before training: 🙂 😐 ☹️ 😜 😠 😟 😊 😎

Feelings after training 🙂 😐 ☹️ 😜 😠 😟 😊 😎

NUTRITION

Meal 1
time eaten: _________

Meal 2
time eaten: _________

Meal 3
time eaten: _________

Meal 4
time eaten: _________

Meal 5
time eaten: _________

Hydration

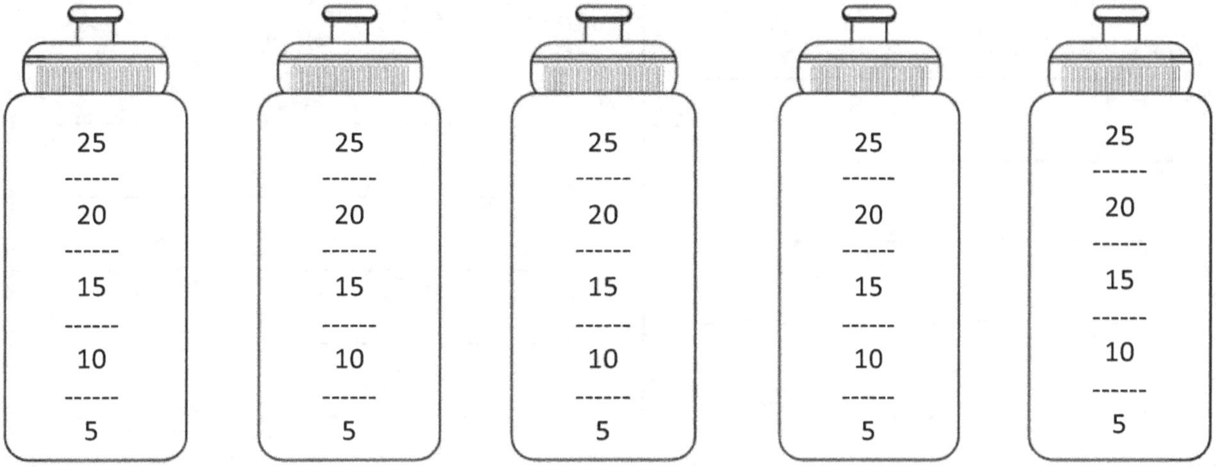

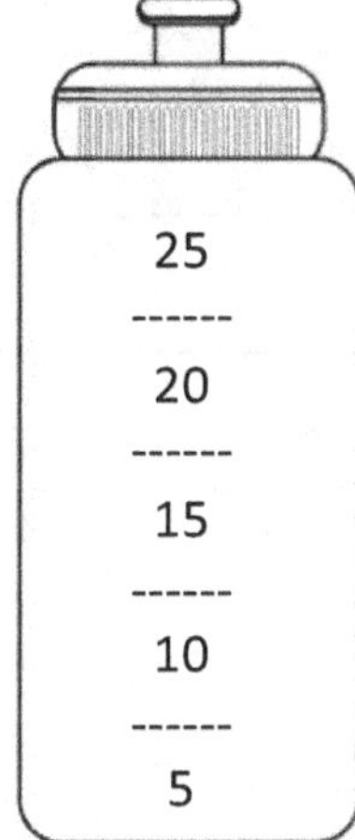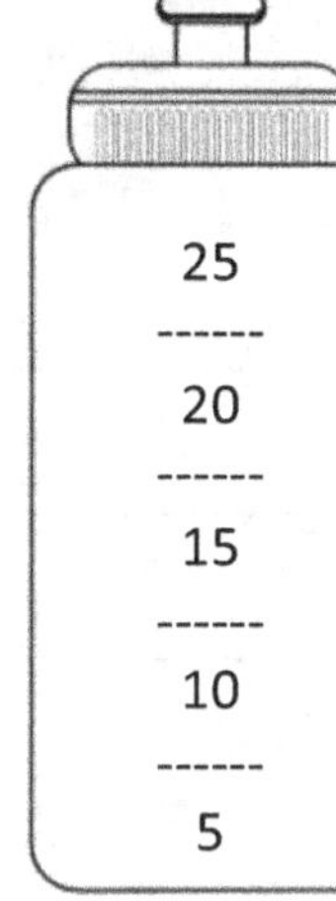

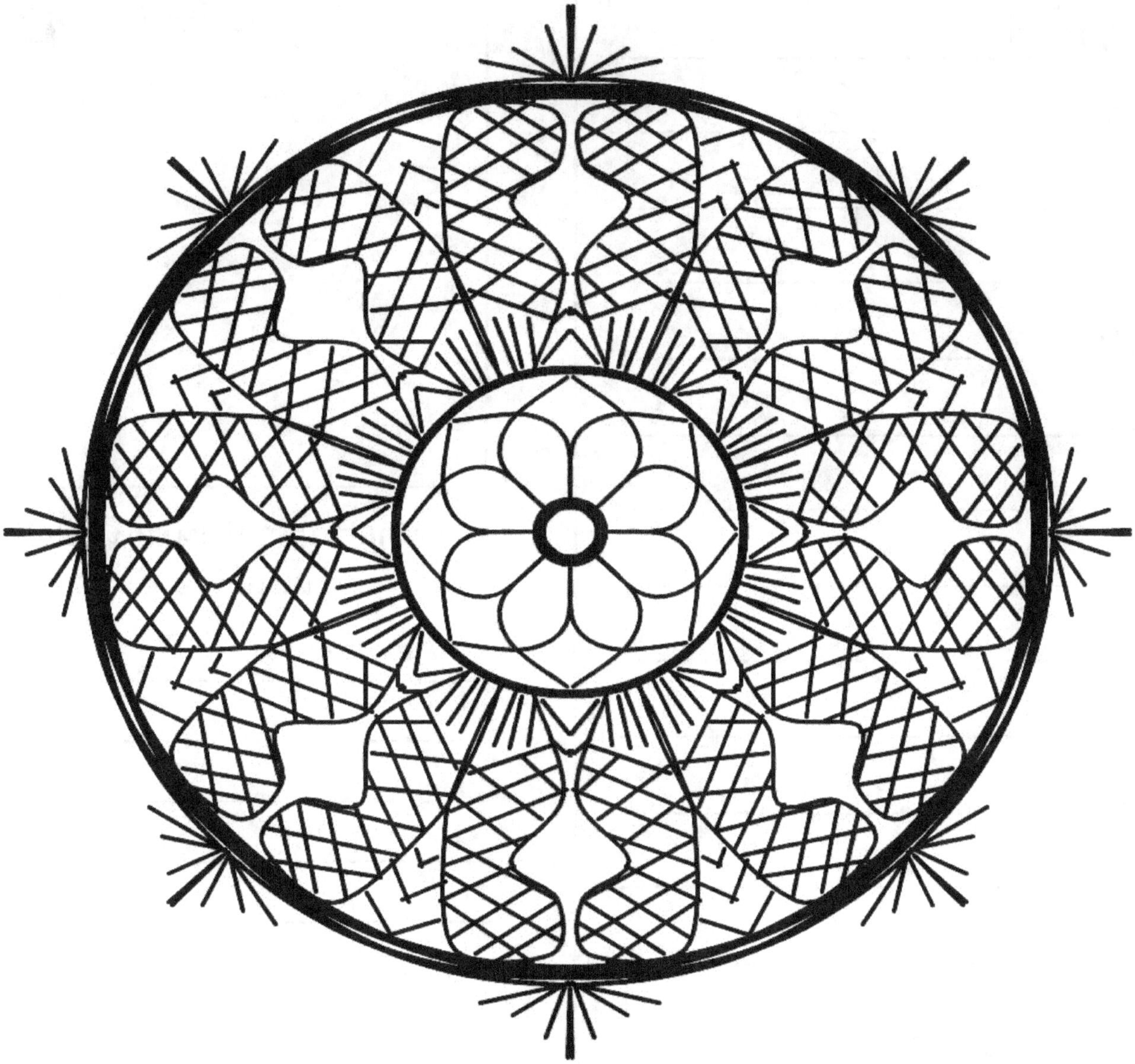

Day Thirty-eight _______

5:00 _______________________

6:00 _______________________

7:00 _______________________

8:00 _______________________

9:00 _______________________

10:00 ______________________

11:00 ______________________

Noon _______________________

1:00 _______________________

2:00 _______________________

3:00 _______________________

4:00 _______________________

5:00 _______________________

6:00 _______________________

7:00 _______________________

8:00 _______________________

9:00 _______________________

10:00 ______________________

11:00 ______________________

Midnight ____________________

top priorities for today 🎯

____

____

____

____

Today's victories 🏆

What does it mean to be alluring?

____

____

____

____

____

____

The *Stella Society* Workout

Exercise	Set 1	Set 2	Set 3	Set 4	Set 5	notes

Time started: ______________ Time ended: ______________

Location: ____

Feelings before training: 🙂 😐 🙁 😜 😣 😟 😊 😎

Feelings after training 🙂 😐 🙁 😜 😣 😟 😊 😎

NUTRITION

Meal 1

time eaten: _________

Meal 2

time eaten: _________

Meal 3

time eaten: _________

Meal 4

time eaten: _________

Meal 5

time eaten: _________

Hydration

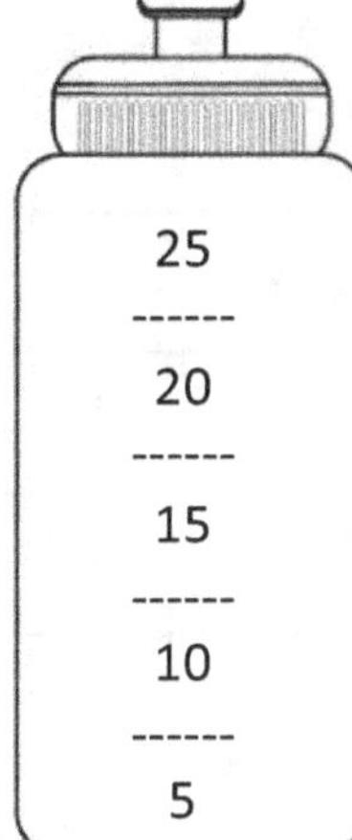

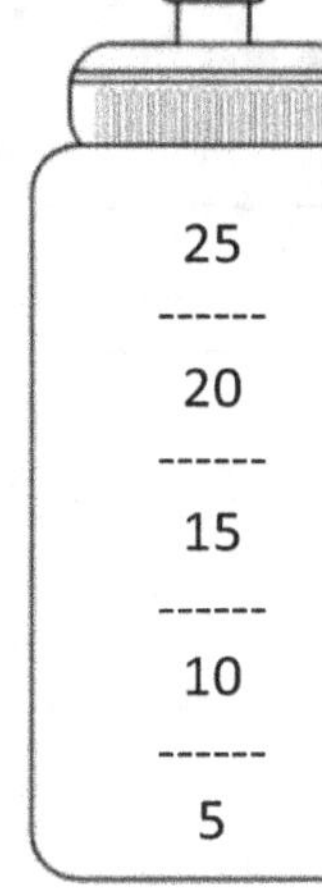

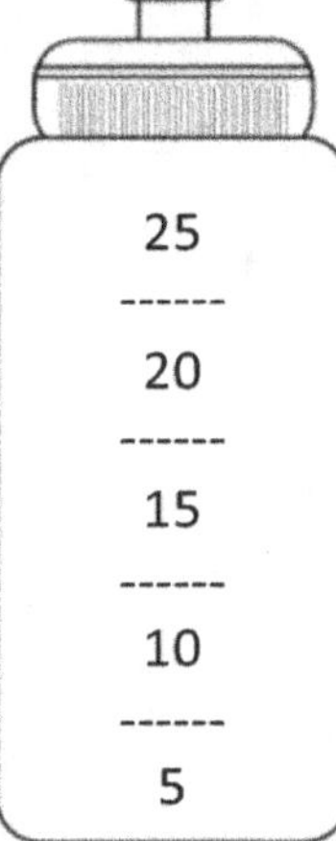

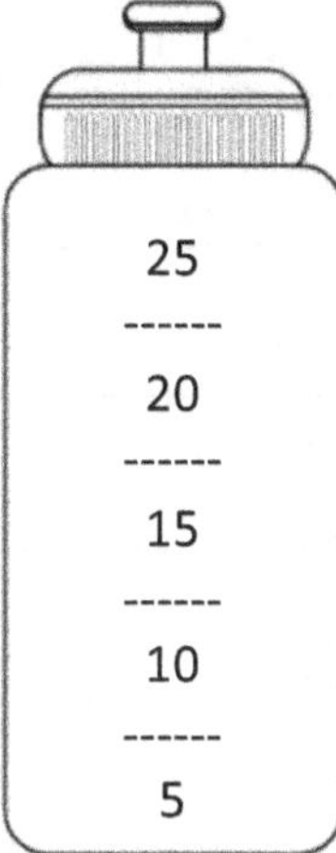

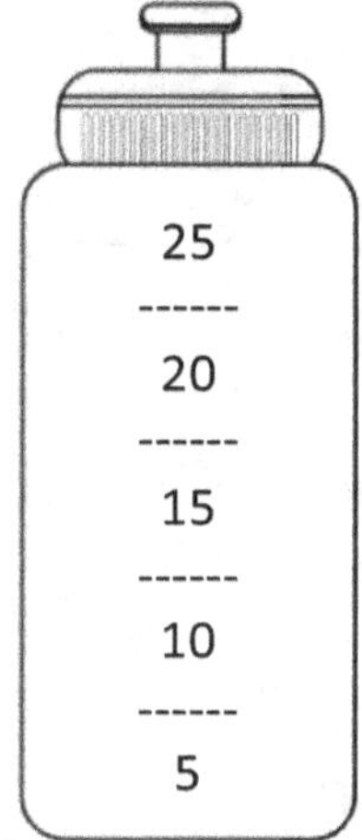

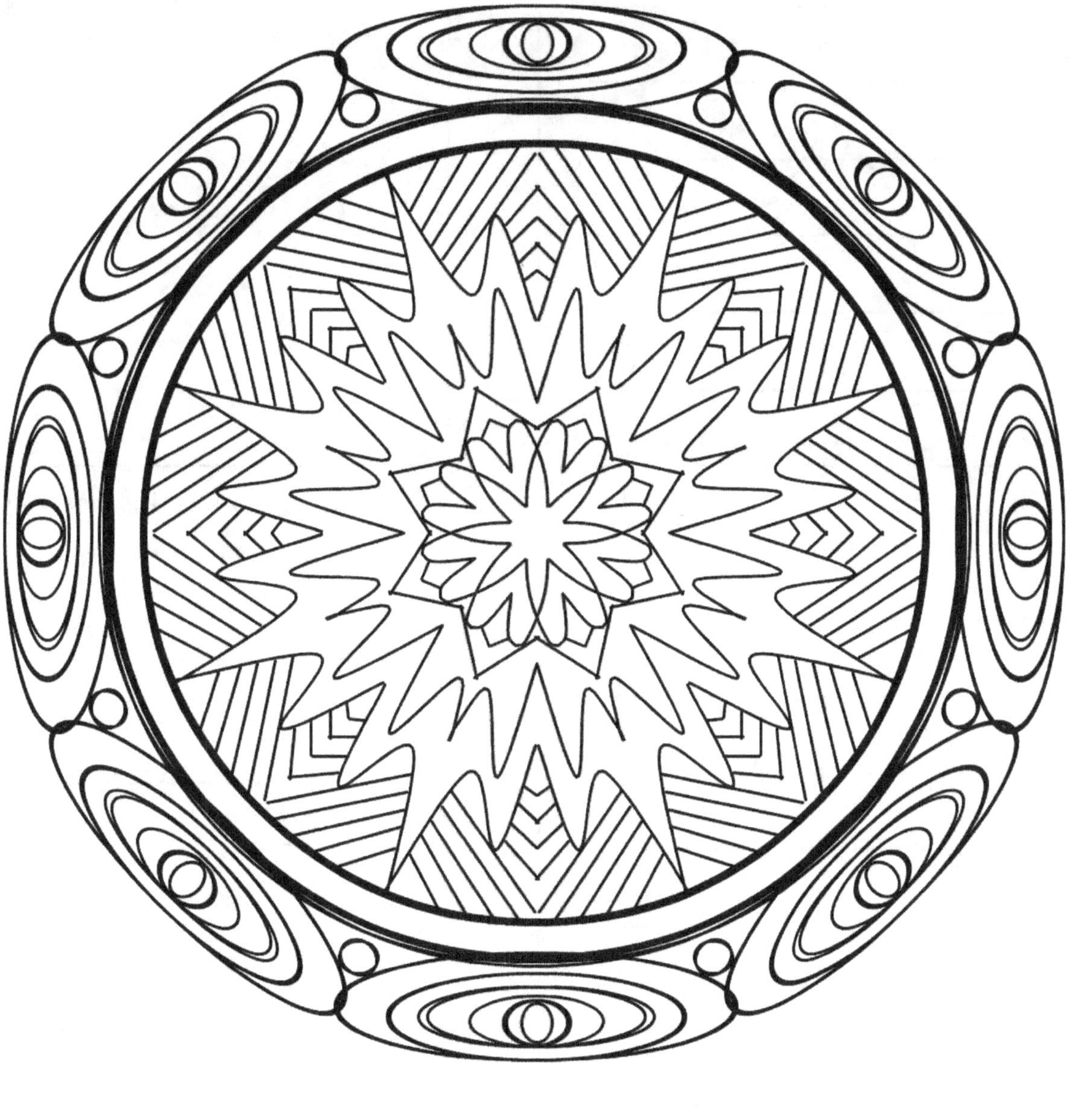

Day Thirty-nine ______

5:00 ______________________

6:00 ______________________

7:00 ______________________

8:00 ______________________

9:00 ______________________

10:00 ______________________

11:00 ______________________

Noon ______________________

1:00 ______________________

2:00 ______________________

3:00 ______________________

4:00 ______________________

5:00 ______________________

6:00 ______________________

7:00 ______________________

8:00 ______________________

9:00 ______________________

10:00 ______________________

11:00 ______________________

Midnight __________________

top priorities for today

Today's victories

How will you be the best
version of you?

The Stella Society Workout

Exercise	Set 1	Set 2	Set 3	Set 4	Set 5	notes

Time started: ______________ Time ended: ______________

Location: ____

Feelings before training: 🙂 😐 🙁 😜 😠 😟 😇 😎

Feelings after training 🙂 😐 🙁 😜 😠 😟 😇 😎

NUTRITION

Meal 1
time eaten: _________

Meal 2
time eaten: _________

Meal 3
time eaten: _________

Meal 4
time eaten: _________

Meal 5
time eaten: _________

Hydration

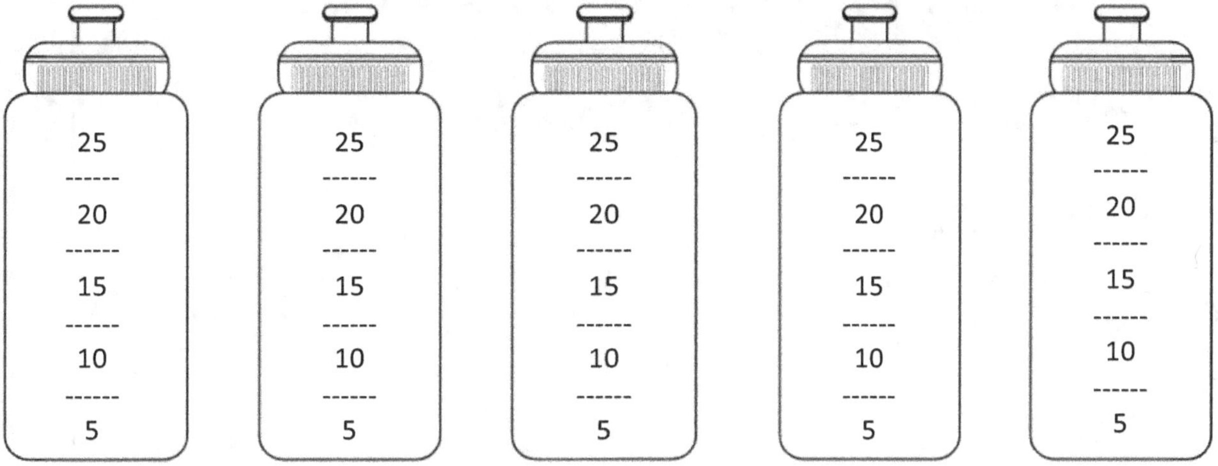

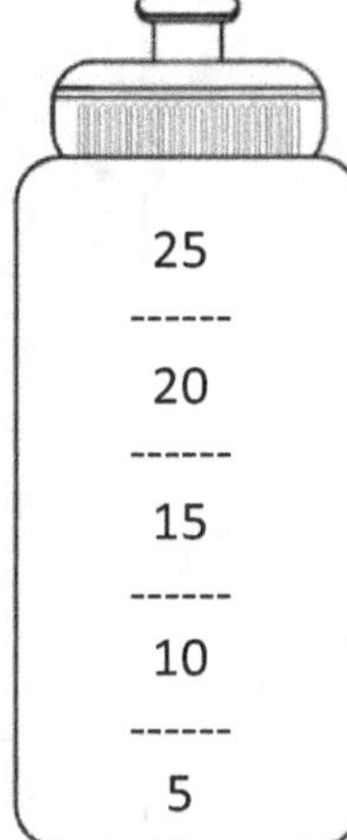
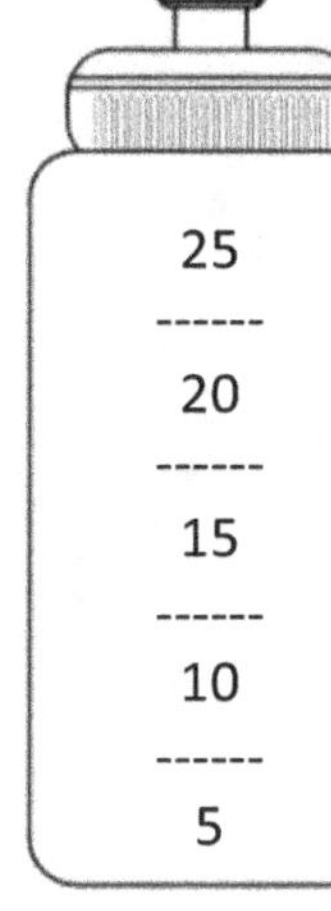
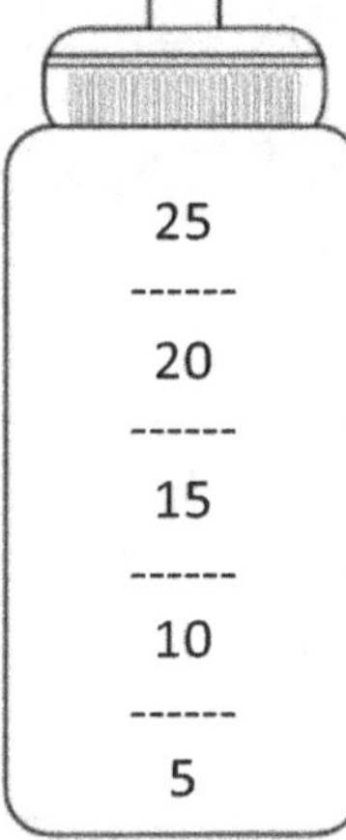

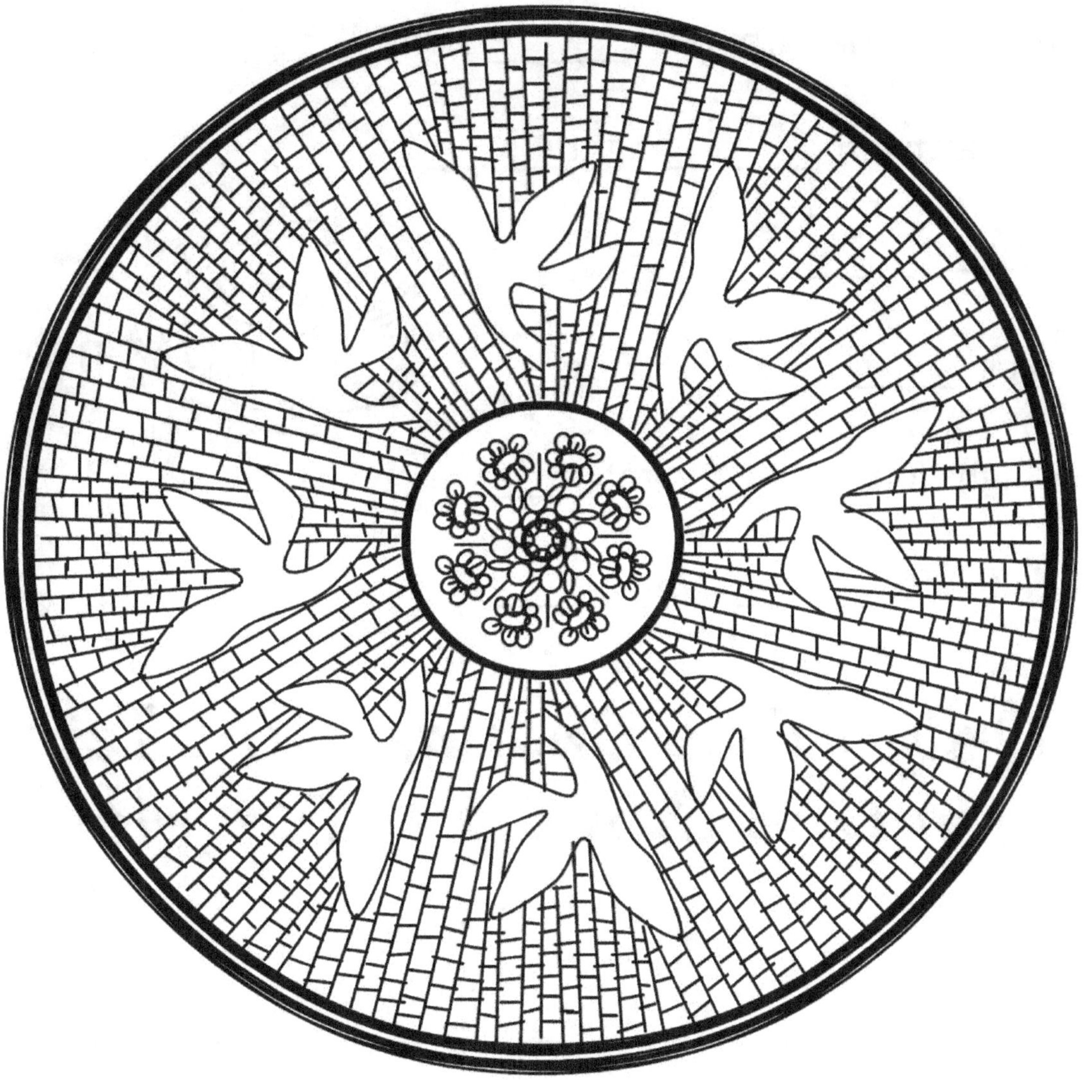

Measurements

DATE: ___________

Weight: _______

Neck _______

Shoulders _______

Chest _______

Bicep / upper arm left _________ right _______

Forearm left _________ right _______

Waist _______

Hips _______

Thighs left _________ right _______

Calf left _________ right _______

*Only I Can Change My Life,
No One Can Do It For Me!*

Day Forty _______

5:00 __________	

5:00 ___________________________
6:00 ___________________________
7:00 ___________________________
8:00 ___________________________
9:00 ___________________________
10:00 __________________________
11:00 __________________________
Noon ___________________________
1:00 ___________________________
2:00 ___________________________
3:00 ___________________________
4:00 ___________________________
5:00 ___________________________
6:00 ___________________________
7:00 ___________________________
8:00 ___________________________
9:00 ___________________________
10:00 __________________________
11:00 __________________________
Midnight _______________________

top priorities for today 🎯

____
____
____
____
____

Today's victories 🏆

Do you believe in magic or miracles?

____
____
____
____
____
____

The Stella Society Workout

Exercise	Set 1	Set 2	Set 3	Set 4	Set 5	notes

Time started: _____________   Time ended: _______________

Location: ____

Feelings before training: 🙂 😐 🙁 😜 😠 😟 😊 😎

Feelings after training 🙂 😐 🙁 😜 😠 😟 😊 😎

NUTRITION

Meal 1

time eaten: _________

Meal 2

time eaten: _________

Meal 3

time eaten: _________

Meal 4

time eaten: _________

Meal 5

time eaten: _________

Hydration

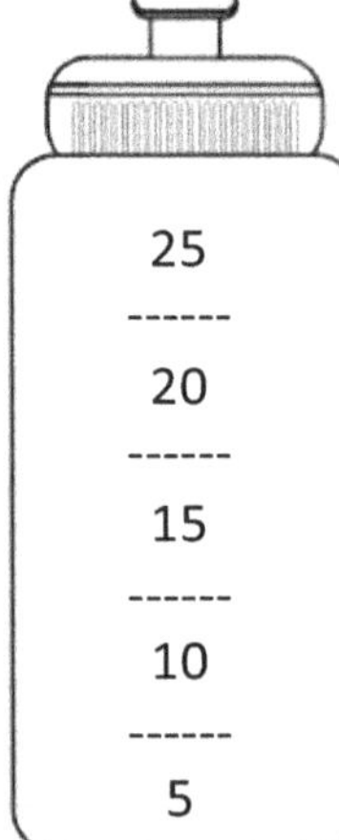 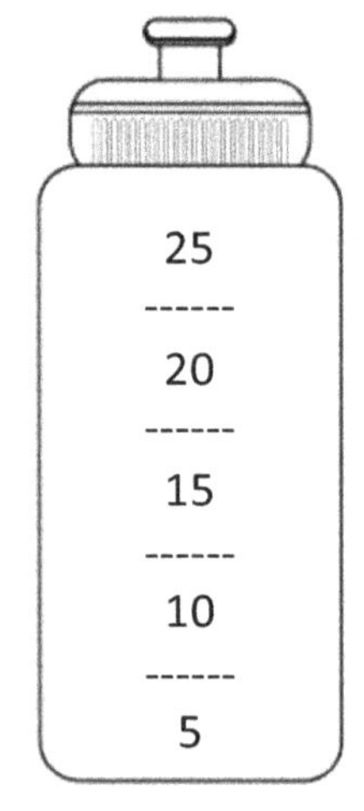 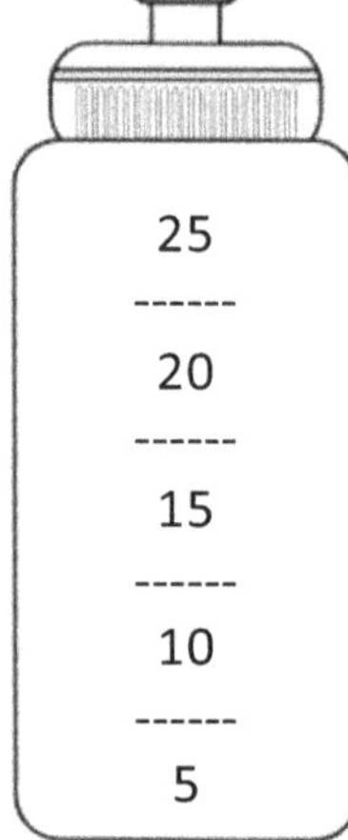 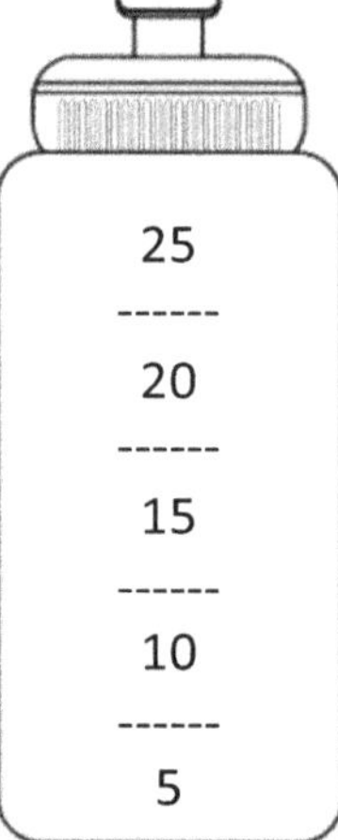 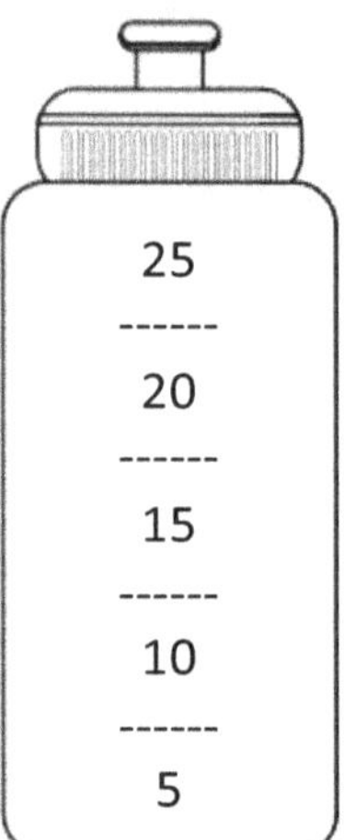

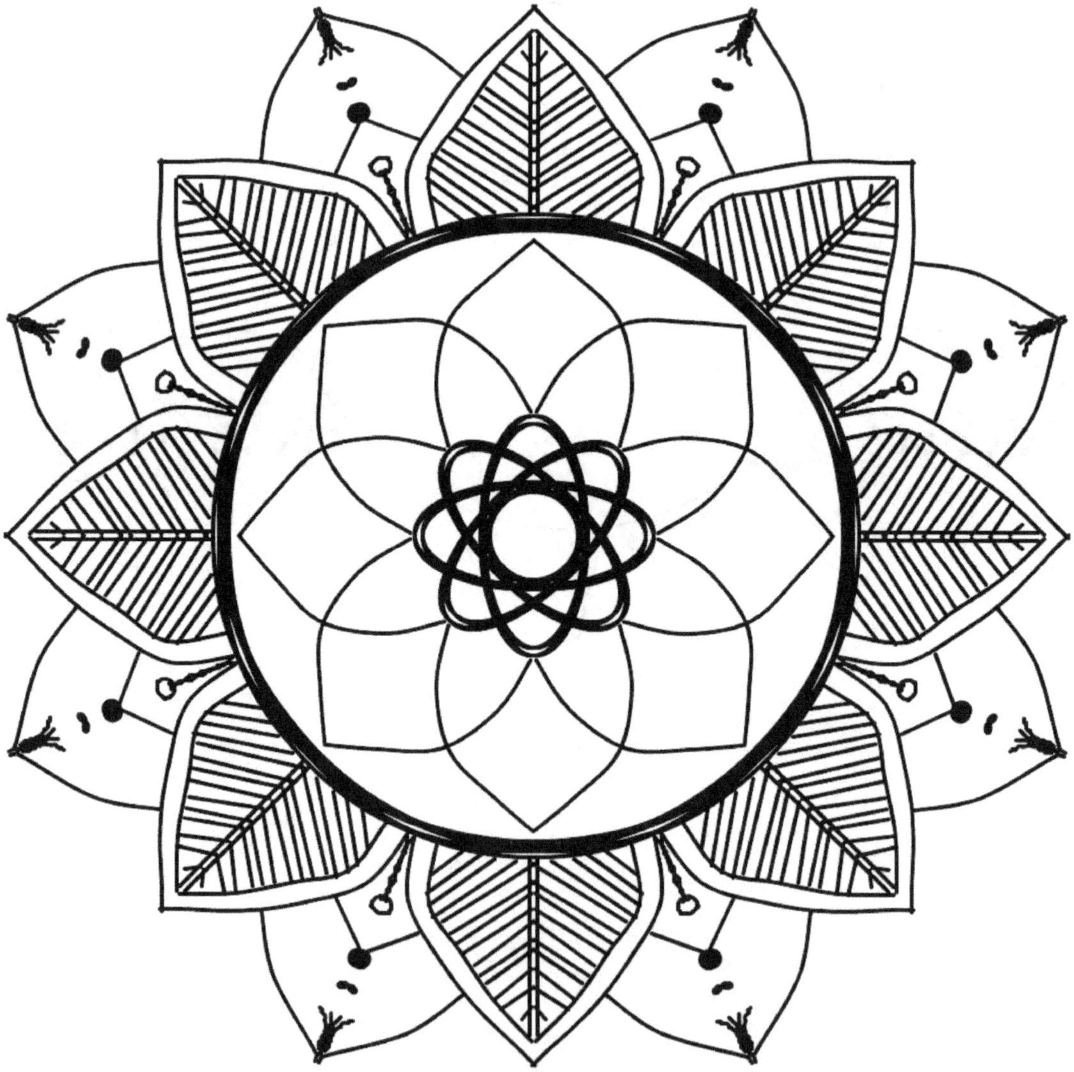

Day Forty-one ______

| | top priorities for today 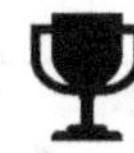 |

5:00 _______________________

6:00 _______________________

7:00 _______________________

8:00 _______________________

9:00 _______________________

10:00 _______________________

11:00 _______________________

Noon _______________________

1:00 _______________________

2:00 _______________________

3:00 _______________________

4:00 _______________________

5:00 _______________________

6:00 _______________________

7:00 _______________________

8:00 _______________________

9:00 _______________________

10:00 _______________________

11:00 _______________________

Midnight ___________________

Today's victories 🏆

What is one thing you
want to do forever?

The Stella Society Workout

Exercise	Set 1	Set 2	Set 3	Set 4	Set 5	notes

Time started: ______________   Time ended: ________________

Location: ____

Feelings before training:

Feelings after training

NUTRITION

Meal 1

time eaten: _________

Meal 2

time eaten: _________

Meal 3

time eaten: _________

Meal 4

time eaten: _________

Meal 5

time eaten: _________

Hydration

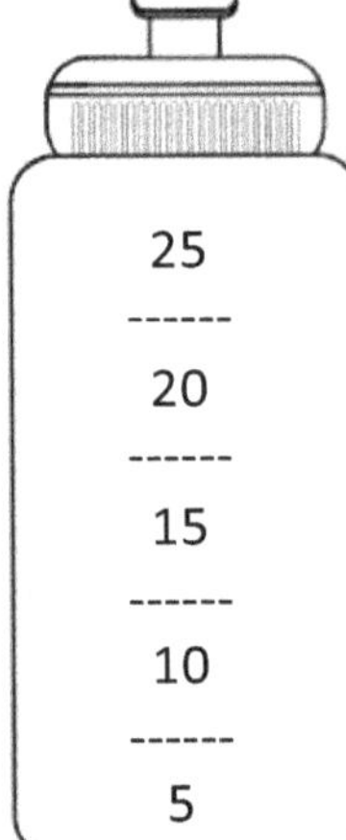

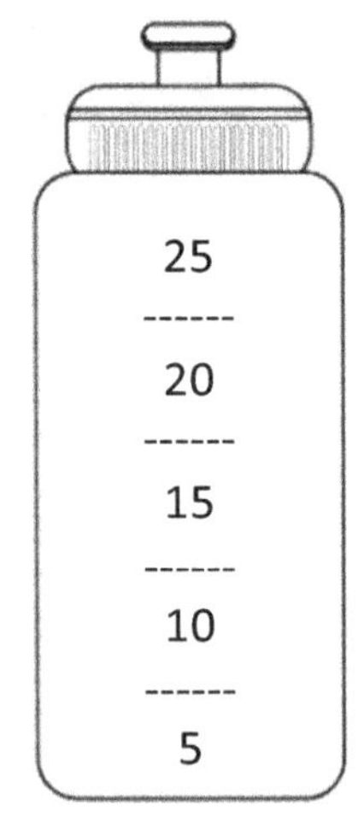

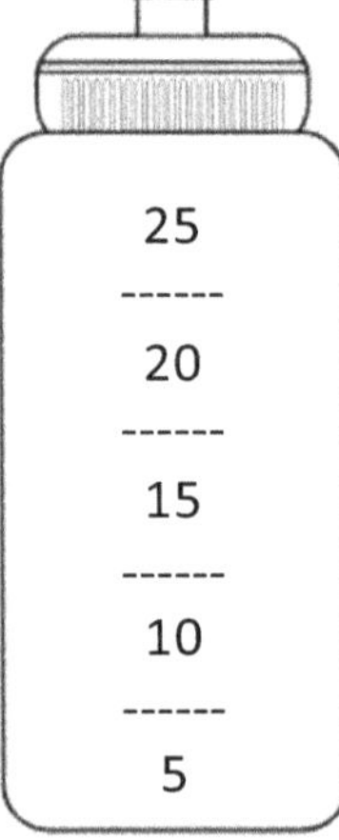

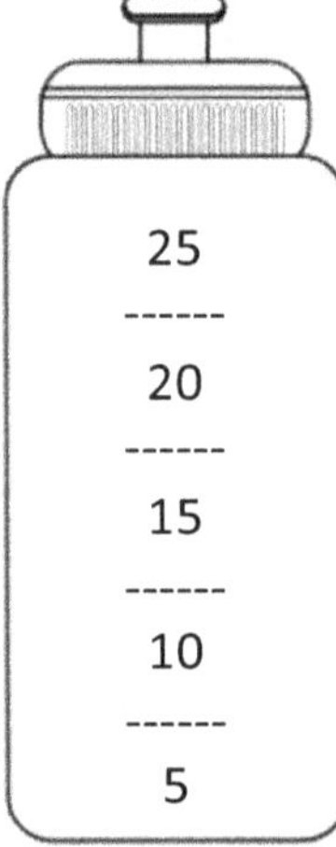

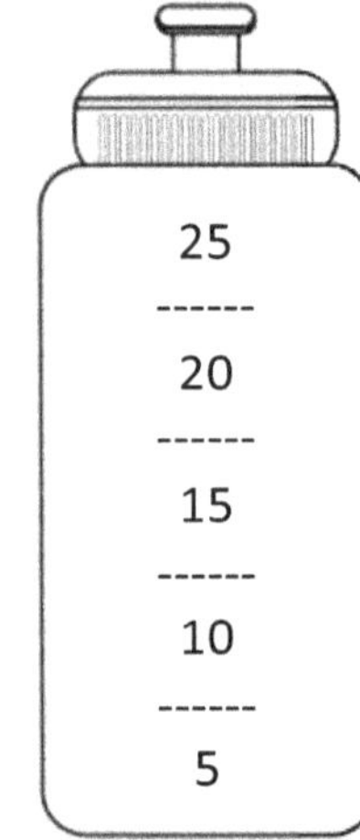

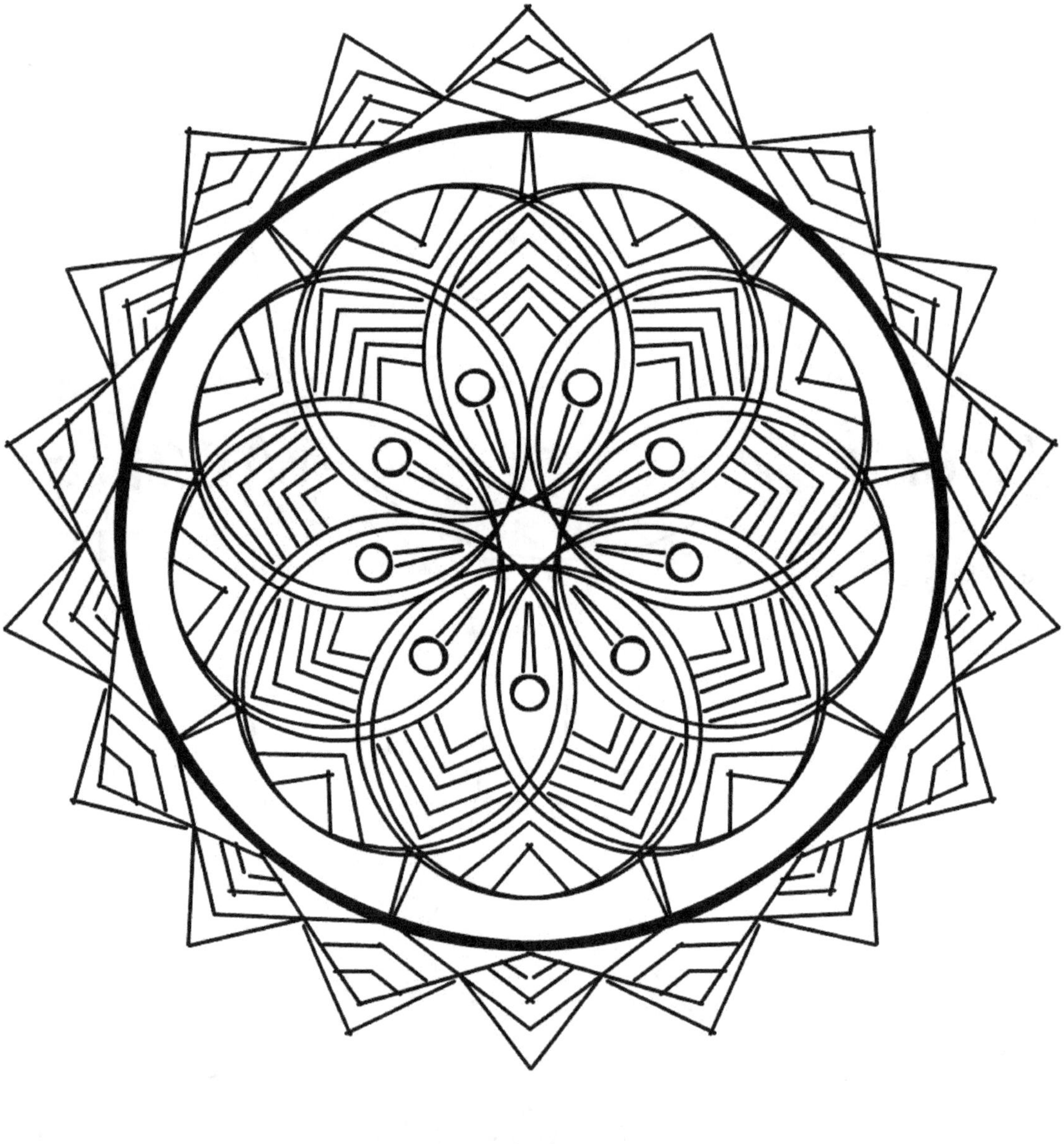

Day Forty-two _______

5:00 _______________________	

5:00 _______________________

6:00 _______________________

7:00 _______________________

8:00 _______________________

9:00 _______________________

10:00 ______________________

11:00 ______________________

Noon _______________________

1:00 _______________________

2:00 _______________________

3:00 _______________________

4:00 _______________________

5:00 _______________________

6:00 _______________________

7:00 _______________________

8:00 _______________________

9:00 _______________________

10:00 ______________________

11:00 ______________________

Midnight ____________________

top priorities for today 

____

____

____

____

____

Today's victories 🏆

What was your biggest
victory in the last 40 days?

____

____

____

____

____

____

____

The *Stella Society* Workout

Exercise	Set 1	Set 2	Set 3	Set 4	Set 5	notes

Time started: ______________   Time ended: ________________

Location: ____

Feelings before training: 😊 😐 🙁 😜 😠 😕 😇 😎

Feelings after training 😊 😐 🙁 😜 😠 😕 😇 😎

NUTRITION

Meal 1

time eaten: _________

Meal 2

time eaten: _________

Meal 3

time eaten: _________

Meal 4

time eaten: _________

Meal 5

time eaten: _________

Hydration

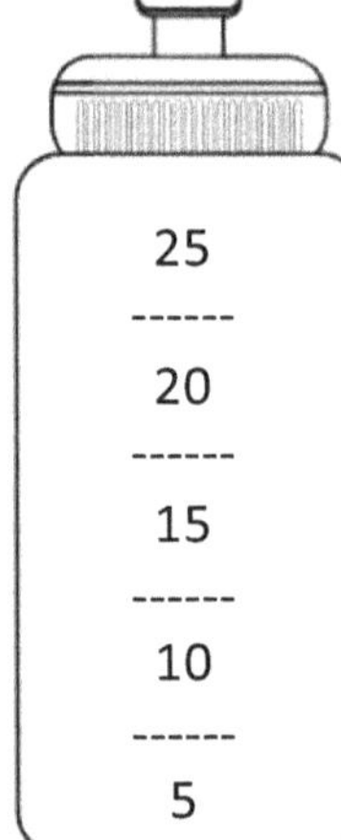
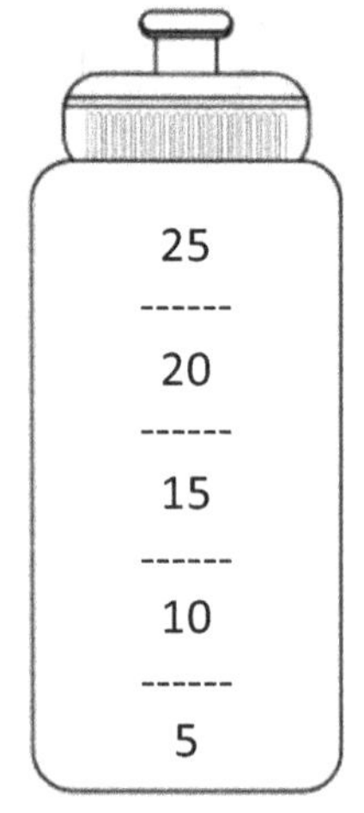
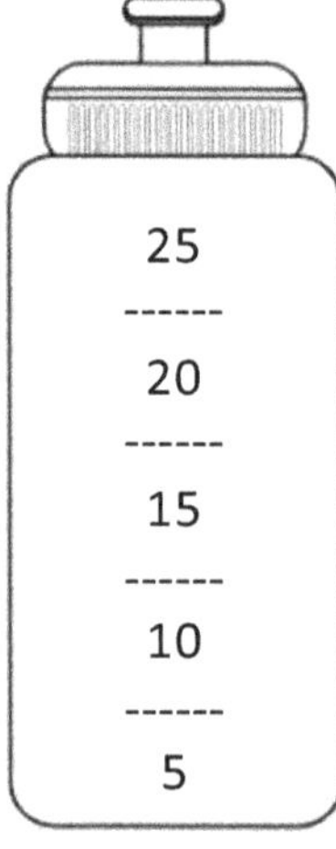
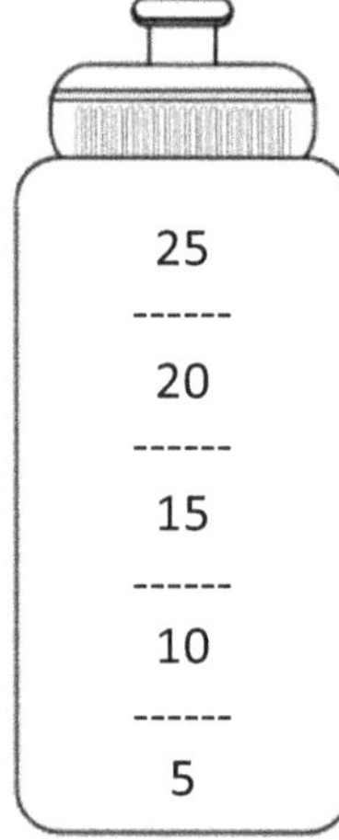
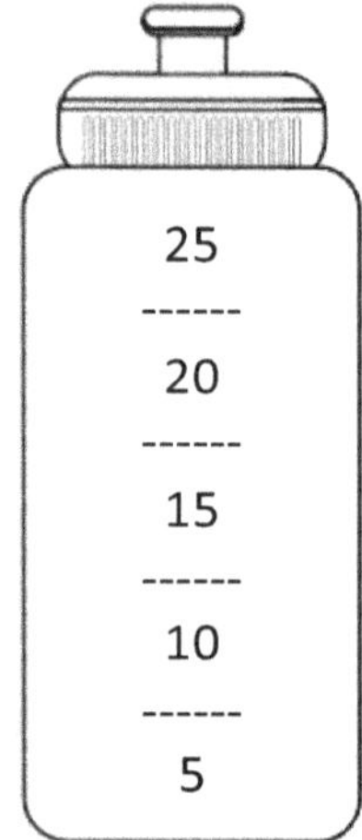

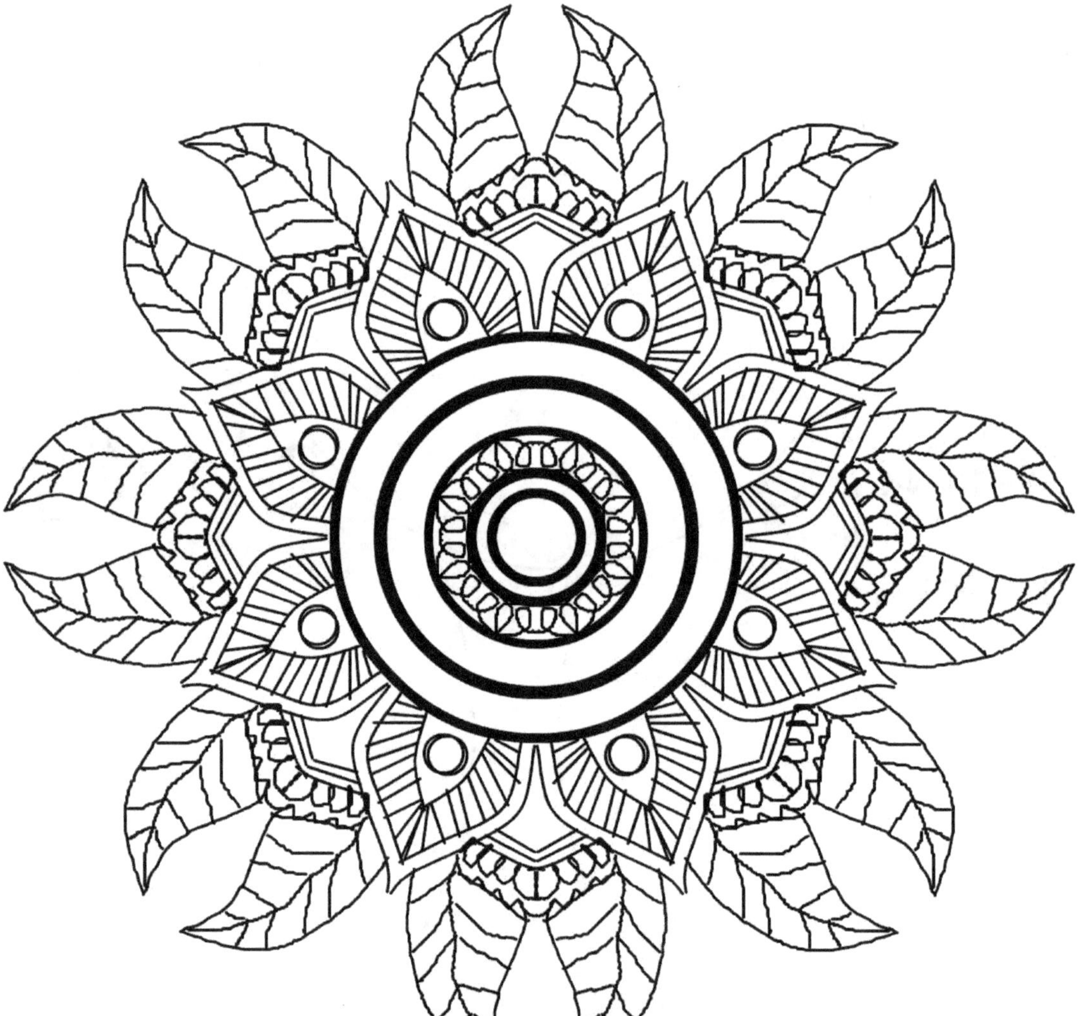

NOW WHAT?